Recent Results in Cancer Research

113

Recent Results in Cancer Research

U. Eppenberger A. Goldhirsch (Eds.)

Endocrine Therapy
and Growth Regulation
of Breast Cancer

With 26 Figures and 17 Tables

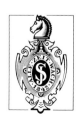

Springer-Verlag
Berlin Heidelberg New York
London Paris Tokyo

Professor Dr. Urs Eppenberger
Laboratorien, Kantonsspital Basel
Universitäts-Frauenklinik
Schanzenstraße 46, 4031 Basel, Switzerland

Priv. Doz. Dr. Aron Goldhirsch
Vice-Primario
Servizio Oncologia Cantonale, Ospedale Civico
6900 Lugano, Switzerland

ISBN 3-540-50456-7 Springer-Verlag Berlin Heidelberg New York
ISBN 0-387-50456-7 Springer-Verlag New York Berlin Heidelberg

Library of Congress Cataloging-in-Publication Data
Endocrine therapy and growth regulation of breast cancer / U. Eppenberger, A. Goldhirsch
(eds.). p. cm. – (Recent results in cancer research : 113) Based on a conference held in 1987.
Includes bibliographies and index.
ISBN 0-387-50456-7 (U.S.: alk. paper): 1. Breast – Cancer – Hormone therapy –
Congresses. 2. Breast Cancer – Endocrine aspects – Congresses. 3. Cancer cells – Growth
Regulation – Congresses. I. Eppenberger, U. II. Goldhirsch, A. (Aron) III. Series
[DNLM: 1. Breast – pathology – congresses. 2. Breast Neoplasms drug therapy –
congresses. 3. Growth Substances – physiology – congresses. 4. Hormones – therapeutic
use – congresses.   W1   RE106P   v. 113 / WP 870 E5555]
RC261.R35   vol. 113   [RC280.B8]   616.99'4 s – dc 19
[616.99'449061]   DNLM/DLC   88-36714

Typesetting, printing, and binding: Appl, Wemding
2125/3140-543210 – Printed on acid-free paper.

Preface

For many physicians and scientists, the transmutation of new scientific discoveries directly from the laboratory bench, the Petri dish or the laboratory animal into improvements in patient care has been a long-standing dream. The fact that, for the most part, realization of this dream remains elusive was recently reflected in a citation by the director of the U.S. National Cancer Institute: "At a time when the rate of progress in many areas is occurring with unprecedented speed ... the need for cross-fertilization is greater than ever ..."

Physicians and basic scientists are, by definition, primarily interested in different - if sometimes related - fields. Thus, laboratory experiments with some practical application for physicians are rare, and clinical studies and their results are often perceived as empirical by basic scientists. The training program of the Swiss Group for Clinical Cancer Research (SAKK) incorporates endeavors at cross-fertilization among disciplines at the clinical-oriented level.

Endocrine therapy for patients with breast cancer is a highly effective treatment modality. It has been shown to delay recurrence and to reduce mortality from the disease, as well as to improve the quality of life of patients whose disease has metastasized. This volume describes experiments related to the use of hormonal agents and to the influence of endocrine and growth factors on the physiology and pathology of breast tissue, both malignant and normal.

The regulation of normal breast tissue and breast cancer growth has been extensively investigated in recent years. Relationships among steroid hormones, growth factors, and growth factor receptors have been defined in relatively simple systems which comprise few interactive phases (e.g., cells of one or two different types and their culture media). To elucidate the actions of hormones and growth factors, as well as their interactions in the most complex system of all - that of the patient with malignant disease - is an ambitious goal.

Remarkably little is known, for instance, about even such simple systems as breast and stromal cells and their interactions, or the mode of communication of cells belonging to the same organ during the various stages of normal development and differentiation. It is possible that some of the mechanisms involved in normal cell growth and in the interaction between epithelial and stromal cells play also a role in the transformation and growth of a malignancy. Unquestionably, illumination of these events will expedite development of improved treatment modalities.

The role of growth factors and their receptors as well as some changes in cell metabolism, function, and growth induced by autocrine and paracrine factors are described in this volume. Ideally, this basic research orientation will serve to stimulate clinically relevant investigations.

Some of the papers presented at the 1987 conference of the SAKK-Educational Symposium held in Lucerne Dec. 4/5, which was sponsored by Ciba-Geigy, F. Hoffmann-La Roche, and Sandoz, have inevitably been updated by subsequent experiments and resultant formulation of new hypotheses. A great deal of the data relates to current issues of considerable significance and has the potential to provide physicians with the impetus to seek new and innovative clinical hypotheses.

Basel/Lugano, December 1988   U. Eppenberger
                                               A. Goldhirsch

Contents

VIII   Contents

List of Contents*

---

* The address of the principal author is given on the first page of each contribution.

[1] Page on which contribution begins.

New Aspects in the Molecular Growth Regulation of Mammary Tumors

U. Eppenberger

Laboratorien, Kantonsspital Basel, Universitäts-Frauenklinik, 4031 Basel, Switzerland

It has been known for many years that there is a close relationship between the growth of human breast cancer and the presence of steroid hormones, such as estrogen and progesterone [1]. With the biochemical discovery of specific receptor proteins for 17 β-estradiol, it was possible to improve the modalities for endocrine therapies. However, despite intensive studies, the molecular mechanisms by which estrogen regulates the growth of breast cancer cells is still poorly understood. With the help of molecular biology we are now starting to understand some of the physiological effects of estrogens. For a few years, we have known that the effect of estrogen is initiated by specific estrogen receptors (ERs) which act as transacting factors on a set of estrogen-inducible genes [2]. The molecular comprehension of estrogen-induced gene transcription will very likely be the key to understand the growth regulation of human breast epithelium cells. Such a transcriptional control is achieved through the interaction of transacting factors with the respective promoter elements located on the DNA. The steroid receptor proteins belong to such a family of regulatory proteins. The ability of these proteins to control gene expression depends on specific ligand binding. The recent cloning of the ER [3] provides the first opportunity to carry out investigations at the molecular level, e.g. the transcription of estrogen-induced proteins. Sequence comparison together with mutational analysis, have defined functional domains in the ER [2, 3]. There is a highly conserved putative DNA-binding domain with two potential DNA-binding fingers which determines the specificity of the ER for the target genes, as well as a region located in the carboxy terminus which confers the specificity for the hormone [2, 3]. There are additional functional regions that are not yet well characterized. These studies have contributed to the understanding of how ERs act on target genes, but both the products of these genes and their involvement in the carcinogenesis of breast epithelium cells and their implication in the growth regulation of human mammary tumors are far from being understood.

Until now we have assumed that estrogen-induced proteins appear to be important in the growth regulation of human breast cancer growth. Several research groups have been able to identify a variety of growth-regulating substances that are secreted in an estrogen-dependent and -independent manner by human mammary tumor cells [4]. As reviewed by Dickson and Lippman, the secretion of IGF-1 (insulin-like growth factor) and α-TGF (transforming growth factor α) were found to be strongly enhanced by estrogen, and are now believed to represent positive autocrine growth factors (GFs). The α-type TGF is known to share 40% homologies with epidermal growth factor (EGF) and may therefore compete with EGF for the EGF receptor (EGF-R). The β-TGF, however, is growth-inhibiting for breast cancer cells, and its secretion seems to be enhanced by antiestrogen (i.e. tamoxifen). Much less is known about the platelet-derived growth factor (PDGF)-related polypeptides which are also secreted by the human breast tumor cell. Although not affecting the growth of breast cancer, they may stimulate stromal proliferation around the tumor, presumably acting as supportive paracrine hormones. Finally, estrogen has also been shown to regulate the levels of certain growth factor receptors, such as EGF-R. According to these findings, one has to accept that there is a GF-dependent growth regulation of human breast cancer.

These GFs interact at the cellular level with specific receptors located at the plasma membrane. They initiate many signals which activate a number of protein kinases such as tyrosine kinase (tyrPK), S6 kinase and the protein kinase PKC. For example, the receptors of EGF/β-TGF, PDGF, insulin and somatomedin C (SM-C) contain a tyrPK activity that is homologous to or reminiscent of the tyrPK activity of viral oncogenes [5]. This tyrPK is activated upon binding of the GF resulting in the autophosphorylation of the respective GF-R and in the phosphorylation of various cellular proteins on tyrosine. Another event closely following the binding of GFs to GF-Rs is the activation of S6 kinase [6]. S6 phosphorylation is believed to be a prerequisite for the initiation of protein synthesis and subsequently DNA synthesis. Finally, in some cases, the activation of GF-Rs results in the hydrolysis of membrane phosphoinositides generating diacylglycerol (DG) and Ca^{2+} which act together to activate the multifunctional PKC, the major receptor for the tumor-promoting phorbol ester [7]. How all these protein kinases are coordinated and translate the GF signal into a mitogenic program remains to be investigated. However, there is general consensus that these different protein kinases play a key regulating role in the transduction of the GR stimulus into a mitogenic signal.

One of the more adverse aspects of breast cancer is that its natural history often involves the transition from an estrogen-responsive tumor to a more aggressive estrogen-unresponsive phenotype. To this date, only the steroid receptors and the lymph-node status are used as valuable prognostic factors in this cancer [8]. Recently, a variety of cellular proto-oncogenes encoding effector molecules of growth regulation have been linked to neoplastic processes based on their homology to retroviral oncogenes. More recently, an additional analogue of the cellular counterpart of the v-*erB* that encodes for the EGF-R has been identified in the human genome. This gene, called *erbB*-2, *HER-2* or C-*neu,* revealed a close structural similarity to the EGF-R [9].

The role of these various proto-oncogenes in the pathogenesis of human malignancies remains unclear. One line of evidence implicating abnormalities of these genes in human diseases is in the association of their amplification with tumor progression in specific cancers. In fact, gene amplification and rearrangement for both the EGF-R and HER-2 have now been identified in a variety of tumor cells [10].

Recently, HER-2 and EGF-R overexpressions have been demonstrated by Slamon et al. [11] and Sainsbury et al. [12] to have greater prognostic value in human breast cancer than most currently used prognostic factors, including the hormonal status, and other disease parameters. The fact that the understanding of the growth regulation of breast tumor has led to such results is encouraging. In summary, these data demonstrate that interdisciplinary efforts may indeed be very valuable. This work discussed in this volume should help disseminate the most up-to-date efforts in the field of breast cancer.

References

1. Edwards DP, Chamness GC, McGuire WL (1979) Estrogen and progesterone receptor proteins in breast cancer. Biochim Biophys Acta 560: 457–486
2. Green S, Chambon P (1986) A superfamily of potentially oncogenic hormone receptors. Nature 324: 615–617
3. Green S, Walter P, Kuma V, Krust A, Bornert JM, Argos P, Chambon P (1986) Human oestrogen receptor cDNA: sequence, expression and homology to v-*erb*-A. Nature 320: 134–139
4. Dickson RB, Lippman ME (1987) Estrogenic regulation of growth and polypeptide growth factor secretion in human breast carcinoma. Endocr Rev 8: 29–43
5. Heldin CH, Westermark B (1984) Growth factors: mechanism of action and relation to oncogenes. Cell 37: 9–20
6. Novak-Hofer I, Martin-Perez J, Thomas G (1986) Epidermal growth factor regulation of S6 phosphorylation during the mitogenic response. In: Nunez J, Denton RM, Dumont JE (eds) Hormones and cell regulation. John Libbey Eurotext, pp 181–197
7. Nishizuka Y (1984) The role of protein kinase C in cell surface signal transduction and tumour promotion. Nature 308: 693–698
8. Millis R (1980) Correlation of hormone receptors with pathological features in human breast cancer. Cancer 46: 2869–2871
9. Schechter AL, Stern FD, Vaidyanathan L, Decker SJ, Jeffrey A, Drebin JA, Greene MI, Weinberg RA (1984) The *neu* oncogene: an *erb*-B-related gene encoding a 185,000-M_r tumour antigen. Nature 312: 513–516
10. Libermann TA, Nusbaum HR, Razon N, Kris R, Lax I, Soreq H, Whittle N, Waterfield MD, Ullrich A, Schlessinger J (1985) Amplification, enhanced expression and possible rearrangement of EGF receptor gene in primary human brain tumours of glial origin. Nature 313: 144–147
11. Slamon DJ, Clark GM, Wong SG, Levin WJ, Ullrich A, McGuire WL (1987) Human breast cancer: correlation of relapse and survival with amplification of the HER-2/*neu* oncogene. Science 235: 177–182
12. Sainsbury JRC, Farndon JR, Needham GK, Malcolm A, Harris AL (1987) Epidermal-growth-factor receptor status as predictor of early recurrence of and death from breast cancer. Lancet i (8547): 1398–1402

In Vitro Cultures of Epithelial Cells from Healthy Breast Tissues and Cells from Breast Carcinomas

U. Regenass[1], D. Geleick[1], E. Curschellas[1], T. Meyer[1], and D. Fabbro[2]

[1] Abteilung für pharmazeutische Forschung, Firma Ciba-Geigy, 4002 Basel, Switzerland
[2] Laboratorien, Kantonsspital Basel, Universitäts-Frauenklinik, 4031 Basel, Switzerland

Introduction

Much of the knowledge concerning the mechanisms involved in the growth regulation of breast cancer comes from the use of cultured cells, particularly cell lines (Lippman et al. 1986; Salomon et al. 1986). During the last few years, techniques have been described which allow the growth directly from patients' tissue of normal human breast epithelial cells (Stampfer et al. 1980; Stampfer 1982; Biran et al. 1983; Taylor-Papadimitriou et al. 1980; Hammond et al. 1984; Briand et al. 1987; Soule and McGrath 1986; Emerman et al. 1987) and of human mammary carcinoma-derived cells (Smith et al. 1981; Simon et al. 1984; Emerman et al. 1987; Petersen and Van Deurs 1987).

A prerequisite for the proper interpretation of growth control mechanisms identified in short-term cultures is the outgrowth of a representative fraction of tumor cells under conditions which preserve the physiological state of the cells comparable to the state in vivo. Therefore, a careful characterization of the cells present in short-term cultures is required. Such an analysis should also reflect the heterogeneity of the tumors at a cellular level.

Culture Systems

The culture media described include both formulations with different types of sera and serum-free formulations. The characteristics of some of these culture conditions are summarized in Tables 1 and 2. In serum-free media, serum is replaced by the addition of defined mitogenic substances including growth factors in addition to bovine serum albumin, bovine pituitary extracts, or high-density lipoproteins. Cholera toxin was added to three of the media (Stampfer 1982; Taylor-Papadimitriou et al. 1983; Soule and McGrath, 1986). The medium described by Stampfer (1982) and designated MM is further characterized by the addition of conditioned media from three different cell lines, whereas the Soule and McGrath (1986) medium is characterized by the use of a low Ca^{++} concentration to allow long-term cell growth.

Culture condition which allow the reproducible growth of a high percentage of normal breast tissue and breast cancer-derived cells might open up the possibility to study breast cancer growth regulation on an individual tumor basis. Such ap-

Recent Results in Cancer Research, Vol. 113
© Springer-Verlag Berlin · Heidelberg 1989

Table 1. Culture conditions for human breast epithelial cells: formulations with serum

Author	Stampfer (1982)	Simon et al. (1984)	Soule, McGrath (1986)	Emerman et al. (1987)
Tissue	Normal/Tumor	Tumor, Metastasis	Normal	Normal/Tumor
DME medium	30%	[a]	47.5%	47.5%
Ham's F-12 medium	30%[b]		47.5%	47.5%
MCDB 170 medium				
β-Estradiol	10^{-9} M	$10^{-8}M$		
Prolactin		50 ng/ml		
L-Thyroxin		$10^{-8}M$		
Insulin	10 µg/ml	3.1 µg/ml	10 µg/ml	5 µg/ml
Hydrocortisone	$2.8 \times 10^{-7}M$	$10^{-7}M$	$1.4 \times 10^{-6}M$	
Transferrin		2.5 µg/ml		
Triiodothyronine	$10^{-8}M$			
Cholera toxin	1 ng/ml		100 ng/ml	
Fibronectin				
Fetuin		5 µg/ml		
Glycyl-L-histidyl -L-lysine		100 ng/ml		
EGF	5 ng/ml		20 ng/ml	
FGF				
Serum	0.5% NBC/FCS	10% FCS	5% HoS	5% HuS
BSA				
BPE				
HDL				
Ca^{++}	~1.4 mM	~2.2 mM	1.05 mM/ 0.06 mM	~1.2 mM
Substrate	Plastic	Plastic	Plastic	Collagen, type I

DME, Dulbecco's modified Eagle's medium; *EGF*, epidermal growth factor; *FGF*, fibroblast growth factor; *BSA*, bovine serum albumin; *BPE*, bovine pituitary extract; *HDL*, high-density lipoprotein; *EA*, essential amino acids; *NEA*, nonessential amino acids; *Vit*, vitamins; *ECM*, extracellular matrix.
[a] Earles salt solution, $2 \times$ MEM vitamins, $2 \times$ EA + $2 \times$ NEA, 4 mM L-glutamine, 1 mM Na pyruvate.
[b] plus HS 74 Int 15% HS 767 Bl 15% HS 578 Bst 9%, conditioned media.

proaches have been initiated recently. Cultures derived from metastasizing human carcinomas have been tested for hormonal growth responses (Simon et al. 1984), and similarly, cultures derived from primary carcinomas, metastases, and healthy breast tissues were analyzed for chemotherapeutic drug sensitivities (Emerman et al. 1987; Smith and Hackett 1987).

Keratin and Vimentin Expression

Keratins and vimentin are intermediate filaments and form part of the cytoskeleton of the vertebrate cell. Keratins are characteristic for epithelial cells, whereas vimentin was found mainly in cells of mesenchymal origin (for review, see Osborn

Table 2. Culture conditions for human breast epithelial cells: serum free formulations

Author	Biran et al. (1983)	Hammond et al. (1984)	Petersen, van Deurs (1987)	Briand et al. (1987)
Tissue	Normal	Normal	Primary carcinoma	Normal
DME medium	50% + NEA		50%[b]	50%
Ham's F-12 medium	50% + Vit.		50%	50%
MCDB 170 medium		100%[a]		
β-Estradiol	$10^{-8}M$		$10^{-8}M$	$10^{-10}M$
Prolactin		1 µg/ml		5 µg/ml
L-Thyroxin				
Insulin	0.2 µg/ml	5 µg/ml	3 µg/ml	0.25 µg/ml
Hydrocortisone	$2.8 \times 10^{-7}M$	$1.4 \times 10^{-7}M$	$1.4 \times 10^{-6}M$	$10^{-6}M$
Transferrin	10 µg/ml	5 µg/ml	25 µg/ml	10 µg/ml
Triiodothyronine			$10^{-9}M$	
Ethanolamine		$10^{-4}M$	$10^{-4}M$	
Phosphoethanolamine		$10^{-4}M$	$10^{-4}M$	
PGE$_1$		$2.5 \times 10^{-8}M$		
Na Selenite	25 ng/ml	in MCDB	2.6 ng/ml	2.6 ng/ml
Ascorbic acid			10 µg/ml	
Dibutyryl c-AMP			$10^{-8}M$	
Cholera toxin				
Fibronectin			100 ng/ml	
Fetuin			20 µg/ml	
Glycyl-L-histidyl -L-lysine				
EGF	25 ng/ml	10/25 ng/ml	100 ng/ml	100 ng/ml
FGF	250 ng/ml			
Serum				
BSA			0.01%	
BPE		70 µg/ml[c]		
HDL	100 µg/ml			
Ca^{++}	~1.05 mM	~2 mM	~1.05 mM	~1.05 mM
Substrate	ECM	Plastic	Collagen, type I	Plastic

Abbreviations see Table 1.
[a] Trace elements included.
[b] Plus trace elements.
[c] Replaces prolactin and PGE$_1$.

and Weber 1986). Keratins represent a family of 19 proteins, and their pattern of expression presumably determines epithelial subtypes and reflects the state of differentiation (Moll et al. 1982, 1983).

Keratin expression in the mammary gland has been reviewed recently (Taylor-Papadimitriou and Lane 1987). The normal mammary gland is a complex epithelial tissue, which expresses keratins typical for simple and stratified epithelia (Moll et al. 1982, 1983). In histologic sections, heterogeneity with respect to the expression of keratins 18 and 19 was demonstrated in epithelial cells of healthy breast tissue and benign lesions, whereas malignant tumors stained homogeneously for both keratins. (Bartek et al. 1985a, 1985b; Nagle et al. 1986). Curschellas et al. (1987) have used a panel of monoclonal antibodies directed to simple epithelia cytokeratins as well as the polyclonal antibody A575 directed to stratified epithelia cytokeratins to characterize the outgrowing cells in the culture medium described by Stampfer et al. (1980). This culture medium allows the growth of epithelial cells from both healthy and malignant tumorous breast tissue, as described previously (Smith et al. 1981). In contrast to tissue sections of carcinomas, only a fraction of the outgrowing cells stained for simple epithelia keratins, whereas cultured cells from healthy breast tissue were all positive for simple epithelia cytokeratins. Since all the cells in both types of cultures stained with the A575 antibody, either a change in the expression of simple epithelia keratins or in the accessibility of these antigens occurred during culturing.

In this context it is interesting to note that the amount of tissue polypeptide antigen (TPA) present in histologic sections of breast carcinomas inversely correlated with the degree of malignancy of the tumor (Döll et al. 1986). The anti-TPA antibody used in this study is known to react with keratins 8, 18, and 19 (Weber et al. 1984). Therefore, simple epithelia keratin expression in vitro could be interpreted as a change in the cytoskeleton towards a physiologic state similar to highly aggressive tumors in vivo.

Vimentin expression has been described for both cultured breast epithelial cells from healthy tissue (Dairkee et al. 1985) and cells of pleural effusions of metastatic breast tumors (Ramaekers et al. 1983). Vimentin was also expressed in all cultures derived from breast carcinomas (Curschellas et al. 1987); however, in tissue sections epithelial cells did not stain positive for vimentin, whereas blood vessels and stromal fibroblasts stained positive and served as an internal control. Azumi and Battifora (1987) showed recently that vimentin was preserved only in a fraction of epithelial or carcinoma cells when tissues were fixed with formaldehyde. In this study, approximately 12% vimentin-positive breast adenocarcinomas were identified. Vimentin filaments in epithelial cells have been interpreted as an in vitro adaptation phenomenon presumably due to the loss of the three-dimensional restriction imposed by the tissue of origin (Ben-Ze'ev 1985; Lane et al. 1983; Osborn et al. 1980). An increase in vimentin expression and a concomitant loss of keratin expression could also correlate with the effect of mitogenic stimuli exerted by the type of culture medium used. Connell and Rheinwald (1983) have shown a change of keratin and vimentin associated with a rapid growth in culture. Furthermore, in kidney epithelial cells, vimentin was expressed in damaged kidneys (Gröne et al. 1987), suggesting that this intermediate filament might be an indicator for regeneration and proliferation in this tissue.

Similarly to cells in the MM medium (Stampfer 1982), we have recently found vimentin to be expressed in cells cultured in the low Ca^{++} medium described by Soule and McGrath (1986). Low Ca^{++} has been demonstrated to uncouple growth from endpoint differentiation in breast epithelial cells (McGrath and Soule 1984), but obviously this does not affect vimentin expression when compared with cultures in other media.

Table 3. Chromosome counts in metaphase spreads

Case	Pas-sage	Medi-um	Chromosome number per metaphase plate																													Total cells	Metaphase plates with chromosome number		
			23	24–32	33	34	35	36	37	38	39	40	41	42	43	44	45	46	47	48	49	50	51	52	53	54	55	56–75	76–91	92	93–138	n	<46 (%)	46 (%)	>46 (%)
Mp 1	T2	MM				2	1					3	2	4	5	6	2	49	2				1						3			80	31.3	61.3	7.5
Mp 2	T2	MM						1					2				2	28												1		34	14.7	82.4	2.9
Mp 5	T2	MM							1								1	19	1												1	23	8.7	82.6	8.7
Mp 12	T1	MM										1			1	1	3	20	1										2		2	31	19.4	64.5	16.1
MaCa 86	T1	MM				2	1						1	1	2	3	3	26	19	7	1			1					1			68	19.1	38.2	42.6
MaCa 87	T1	MM												3	2	1	3	16	1	1	1								4			32	28.1	50.0	21.9
MaCa 88	T1	MM											2	1	3	6	13	6	2	1									3	1		38	65.8	15.8	18.4
MaCa 89	T1	MM												1	1	2	3	24	1													32	21.9	75.0	3.1
MaCa 86	T1	MG													2	2	13	8	5	3	1											34	50.0	23.5	26.5
MaCa 87	T1	MG									1				2	2	6	10	3												1	1	29	44.8	34.5	20.7
MaCa 88	T1	MG						1	1	1						1	2	16	1									2	1			28	28.6	57.1	14.3
MaCa 89	T1	MG												2	1	4	7	3	1	1									4			23	60.9	13.0	26.1

Cytogenetic Studies

To determine cytogenetic alterations in breast cancer, short-term cultures offer an alternative to direct chromosomal preparations (Rodgers et al. 1984; Hill et al. 1987) and established cell lines (Satya-Prakash et al. 1984). The MM medium has been preferentially applied for this purpose to primary breast cancer (Smith et al. 1985a; Wolman et al. 1985). These studies revealed predominantly diploid cells for primary breast cancer with a low frequency of metaphases with nonclonal chromosomal aberrations. It has therefore been speculated (Trent 1985; Smith et al. 1985b) that the culture conditions might favor the growth of diploid cells and select against highly aneuploid tumor cells. Geleick et al. (1988) have recently reinvestigated the cytogenetics of primary breast cancer using a approach similar to that of Wolman et al. (1985), but with some modifications (e.g., no separation of single cells from cell clumps after digestion, analysis of an increased number of metaphases). It was possible to demonstrate that (a) carcinoma derived cultures were characterized by a high degree of chromosomal instability (losses and gains of chromosomes) and an increased number of methaphases in the hyperdiploid range, (b) in nine out of ten tumors, cells with 46 chromosomes turned out to have chromosomal aberrations in up to 57% of the cells (pseudodiploidism), and (c) in ten malignant tumors analyzed karyotypically, chromosomal aberrations and/or marker chromosomes could be identified, whereas in cultures derived from healthy tissues only occasional chromosome gains and losses were seen. This study supports and extends the findings of Wolman et al. (1985) and demonstrates that carcinoma-derived cultures can be unequivocally distinguished from cultures derived from healthy breast tissue.

In order to study the possibility of the selective growth of a particular cell population in the MM medium, the modal chromosome numbers of four carcinomas grown in the low Ca^{++} medium (Soule and McGrath 1986) were compared with the results obtained in the MM medium. Differences between the two culture media were obtained for individual tumors in the amount of metaphases with particular chromosome numbers (Table 3). When the relative frequencies of metaphases with a particular chromosome number were considered, the curves from breast cancer-derived cultures in both media were similar to but significantly different from cultures of normal breast epithelial cells (Fig. 1). Hyperdiploid cells were present in both culture media in similar amounts.

The modal chromosome distribution of individual tumors (Table 3) suggests that different cell populations might be present in the two media at the time of chromosomal analysis. A similar finding was made when chromosomes were analyzed from the same tumor sample but a different time points after culture initiation (Geleick et al. 1988). In this study, the largest cell population in carcinomas was truly diploid, and the majority of chromosomal aberrations were nonclonal. This finding would be in agreement with the hypothesis of karyotypic instability in primary breast carcinomas and a major fraction of cells in the diploid state.

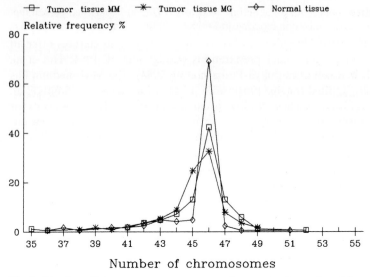

Fig. 1. Number of chromosomes were counted per metaphase plate. Metaphases with a given number of chromosomes from all normal cultures or malignant tumor-derived cultures in a particular culture medium were added and expressed relative to the total number of cells analyzed. Data for normal tissue and malignant tumor tissue-derived cultures in MM medium are from Geleick et al. (1988). *MM*, medium described by Stampfer (1982); *MG*, medium described by Soule and McGrath (1986)

Receptor Determinations and Protein Kinase Activities

Mammary carcinoma (Ma Ca)-derived cells and normal cells derived from mammoplasty (MP) were expanded in MM medium for receptor and protein kinase determinations. As demonstrated in Table 4, all cultures were positive for progesterone receptors (PGR), indicating that they have functional estrogen receptors (ER). At the time of determination, the binding sites for ER might have been masked in two Ma Ca (32, 52) and in the MP-derived cultures. Three tumors (Ma Ca 30, 35, 52) were determined as ER/PGR negative by the receptor determination in biopsies, but positive when analyzed in the cell cultures. This finding is not surprising, since large variations in ER levels have been demonstrated in different areas of breast tumors (van Netten et al. 1985).

Epidermal growth factor (EGF) is an important growth-promoting factor for breast epithelial cells (Hammond et al. 1984). It has been demonstrated recently that the EGF-R content correlates inversely with the ER/PGR content (Fabbro et al. 1986). As shown in Table 4, of our Ma Ca cultures characterized by high ER/PGR content only one (Ma Ca 29) had a low number of EGF receptors. Whether the EGF present in the culture medium in addition to growth factors added by the conditioned media allowed the preferential growth of tumor cells with high numbers of EGF receptors remains unknown.

Protein kinase C (PKC) activity plays an important role in the multiple signalling pathways in response to mitogenic stimuli (for review, see Nishizuka 1986;

Table 4. Estrogen receptors *(ER)*, progesterone receptors *(PGR)* and epidermal growth factor receptors *(EGF-R)* determined in biopsies and primary cultures of mammary carcinomas *(Ma Ca)* and normal *(MP)* tissue

Specimen	Biopsies (f mol/mg protein)		Cell cultures (p mol/mg DNA)		
	ER[a]	PGR[a]	ER[a]	PGR[a]	EGF-R[b]
Ma Ca 27	510 ± 48	94 ± 9	3.08	14.4	3.0
Ma Ca 29	117 ± 8	425 ± 29	3.03	6.7	0.4
Ma Ca 30	9 ± 3	8 ± 4	0.5	11.8	3.0
Ma Ca 32	123 ± 12	163 ± 20	0	15.6	4.0
Ma Ca 35	6 ± 3	0	1.5	41.6	2.5
Ma Ca 37	282 ± 23	179 ± 21	1.1	48.3	2
Ma Ca 52	4 ± 1	0	0	6.4	6.0
MP 2	n.t.	n.t.	0	15	12.8
MCF-7 line	n.t.	n.t.	~0.9- ~3.3[c]	~0.6- ~2.6[c]	~0.2[c]
T47-D line	n.t.	n.t.	~0.7[c]	~22.1[c]	~0.5[c]
MDA-MB-231 line	n.t.	n.t.	0	0	~6.0[c]

n.t., not tested or no data available.
[a] ER and PGR were determined as described by Taylor et al. (1984).
[b] EGF receptors were determined as described by Fabbro et al. (1986).
[c] Recalculated under the assumption that 1 μg DNA corresponds to ~35000 cells based on data presented previously (Fabbro et al. 1986).

Table 5. Protein kinase activities in primary cultures of mammary carcinomas

Specimen	PKC[a] Total (units/mg protein)[c]	PKA[b] Total (units/mg protein)[c]
Ma Ca 27	140	276
Ma Ca 29	190	297
Ma Ca 30	1035	632
Ma Ca 32	124	288
Ma Ca 35	229	326
Ma Ca 37	106	291
Ma Ca 52	221	444
MCF-7 line	520	446

[a] Protein kinase C, determined as described by Fabbro et al. (1985a).
[b] C-AMP-dependent protein kinase, determined as described by Fabbro et al. (1985b).
[c] One unit is defined as the amount of enzyme transferring one pmol ^{32}P per min to the substrate.

Rozengurt 1986). With one exception (Ma Ca 30), all our mammary carcinoma-derived cultures exhibited low PKC levels (Table 5). This might be due to the low mitotic activity in cultures and the partial senescence of the cells after culture expansion. In particular, low PKC levels have been described in ER/PGR positive tumor lines (Fabbro et al. 1986). Ma Ca 30 exhibited an unusually high PKC activity. Cyclic-AMP-dependent protein kinase levels did not differ dramatically among different cultures and were within the range of previously published data (Fabbro et al. 1986).

Histopathologically, Ma Ca 30 was described as a solid, partially dissolute carcinoma. The tumor was found in fibrous stromal tissue and might represent a local recurrence of an invasive duct breast cancer. When cultured in MM medium, fibroblastoid (spindle-shaped) cells grew out of cell clumps (Fig. 2). These cells were keratin negative, vimentin positive, and characterized by an unusually high initial growth rate. Ma Ca 30 displayed hormone and EGF receptors (Table 4). Cytogenetically, these cells were characterized by a numerical chromosome distribution typical for carcinomas and by chromosomal aberrations (Geleick et al. 1988). Morphologically similar cells have been described previously as a differentiation product of the human breast carcinoma line PMC 42 (Whitehead et al. 1983). In this case, the spindle-shaped cells also lacked the expression of keratin.

Spindle-shaped cells in breast tissue-derived cultures were also described for carcinosarcoma cells (HS578T) and myoepithelial cells (HS578Bst) (Hackett et al. 1977). Besides vimentin, some of the Hs578Bst cells also expressed keratins (Curschellas et al. 1987).

Most likely Ma Ca 30-derived cells represent a population of tumor-derived fibroblasts with a foetal-like phenotype and karyotypic abnormalities (for review, see Schor and Schor 1987).

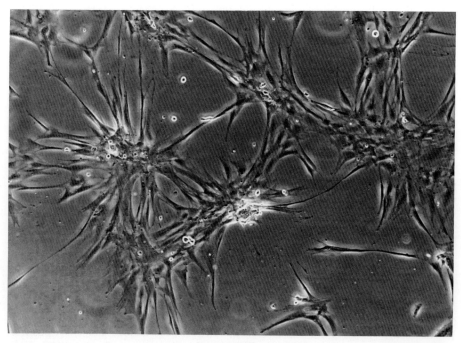

Fig. 2. Ma Ca 30, 5 days after culture innoculation in MM medium. *MM,* medium described by Stampfer (1982)

Conclusions

1. Several culture media which allow the growth of normal human breast epithelial cells and cells derived from primary breast carcinomas have recently been described. Short-term cultures can be obtained from a majority of tissue samples in MM medium (Stampfer 1982) and the low Ca^{++} medium (Soule and McGrath 1986) irrespective of the type of origin.
2. Truly epithelial cells were obtained in MM and low Ca^{++} medium, as shown by the expression of keratins typical for stratified and simple epithelia. Rare exceptions in malignant tumor-derived cultures were identified. When antibodies directed to simple epithelia keratins were used, the staining pattern in vitro differed when compared with that of tissue sections. Similarly, cells in vitro expressed high amounts of vimentin not found to the same degree in tissue sections. The physiological consequences of these differences are as yet unknown.
3. Cell populations derived from carcinomas can be distinguished from cultured cells derived from healthy breast tissue on a cytogenetic basis. The karyotypic instability in cells derived from malignant tumors was unique and not found in normal cells.
4. The cells in culture do express variable levels of receptors for estrogen, progesterone, EGF and the enzyme PKC. It has not yet been possible to establish the correlation among receptors and PKC levels as described for cell lines and biopsies (Fabbro et al. 1986) in these short-term cultures.

Short-term cultures of human primary breast cancer cells should now offer the possibility of analyzing the growth control mechanisms of this disease in comparison with those of normal breast epithelial cells.

References

Azumi N, Battifora H (1987) The distribution of vimentin and keratin in epithelial and non-epithelial neoplasms. Am J Clin Pathol 88: 286–296

Bartek J, Taylor-Papadimitriou J, Miller N, Millis R (1985a) Patterns of expression of keratin 19 as detected with monoclonal antibodies in human breast tissues and tumors. Int J Cancer 36: 299–306

Bartek J, Durban EM, Hallowes RC, Taylor-Papadimitriou J (1985b) A subclass of luminal epithelial cells in the human mammary gland, defined by antibodies to cytokeratins. J Cell Sci 75: 17–33

Ben-Ze'ev A (1985) The cytoskeleton in cancer cells. Biochim Biophys Acta 780: 197–212

Biran S, Horowitz AT, Fuks Z, Vlodavsky I (1983) High-density lipoprotein and extracellular matrix promotes growth and plating efficiency of normal human mammary epithelial cells in serum-free medium. Int J Cancer 31: 557–566

Briand P, Petersen OW, van Deurs B (1987) A new nontumorigenic human breast epithelial cell line isolated and propagated in chemically defined medium. In Vitro Cell Dev Biol 23: 181–188

Connell ND, Rheinwald JG (1983) Regulation of the cytoskeleton in mesothelial cells: reversible loss of keratin and increase in vimentin during rapid growth in culture. Cell 34: 245–253

Curschellas E, Matter A, Regenass U (1987) Immunolocalization of cytoskeletal elements in human mammary epithelial cells. Eur J Cancer Clin Oncol 23: 1517–1527

Dairkee SH, Blayney CM, Asarnow DM, Smith S, Hackett AJ (1985) Early expression of vimentin in human mammary cultures. In Vitro Cell Dev Biol 21: 321–327

Döll S, Klinge U, Schauer A, Bandlow G, Mross K (1986) Immunhistologischer Nachweis der TPA-Expression bei gut- und bösartigen Tumoren der Mamma. In: Wüst G (ed) Tumormarker. Steinkopff-Verlag, Darmstadt, pp 210–212

Emerman JT, Fiedler EE, Tolcher AW, Rebbeck PM (1987) Effects of defined medium, fetal bovine serum, and human serum on growth and chemosensitivities of human breast cancer cells in primary culture: inference for in vitro assays. In Vitro Cell Dev Biol 23: 134–140

Fabbro D, Jungmann AR, Eppenberger U (1985a) Subcellular distribution of protein kinase C of GH3 cells: quantitation and characterization by polyacrylamide gel electrophoresis. Archs Biochem Biophys 239: 102–111

Fabbro D, Bally K, Koudelka G, Jungmann RA, Eppenberger U (1985b) cAMP-dependent protein kinases in rat pituitary GH3 cells. J Cyclic Nucleotide Protein Phosphor Res 10: 31–42

Fabbro D, Wyss R, Borner C, Regazzi R (1986) Epidermal growth factor receptor and calcium/phospholipid-dependent protein kinase activities in human mammary tumor cells. In: Eppenberger U, Fabbro D, Schäfer P (eds) Endocrine therapy of breast cancer. Karger, Basel, pp 33–44. Contribution to oncology, vol 23

Geleick D, Mueller HJ, Matter A, Torhorst J, Regenass U (1988) Cytogenetics of breast cancer. In preparation

Gröne HJ, Weber K, Gröne E, Helmchen U, Osborn M (1987) Coexpression of keratin and vimentin in damaged and regenerating tubular epithelia of the kidney. Am J Pathol 129: 1–8

Hackett AJ, Smith HS, Springer LE, Owens RB, Nelson-Rees WA, Rigg JL, Gardner MB (1977) Two syngeneic cell lines from human breast tissue: the aneuploid mammary epithelial (Hs578T) and the diploid myoepithelial (Hs578Bst) cell lines. J Natl Cancer Inst 58: 1795–1806

Hammond SL, Ham RG, Stampfer MF (1984) Serum-free growth of human mammary epithelial cells: rapid clonal growth in defined medium and extended serial passage with pituitary extract. Proc Nat Acad Sci USA 81: 5435–5439

Hill SM, Rodgers CS, Hulten MA (1987) Cytogenetic analysis in human breast carcinoma. II. Seven cases in the triploid/tertraploid range investigated using direct preparation. Cancer Genet Cytogenet 24: 45–62

Lane EB, Hogan BLM, Kurkinen M, Garrels JI (1983) Co-expression of vimentin and cytokeratins in parietal endoderm of early mouse embryo. Nature 303: 701–704

Lippman ME, Dickson RB, Bates S, Knabbe C, Huff K, Swain S, McManaway M, Bronzert D, Kasid A, Gelmann PE (1986) Autocrine and paracrine growth regulation of human breast cancer. Breast Cancer Res Treat 7: 59–70

McGrath CM, Soule HD (1984) Calcium regulation of normal human mammary epithelial cell growth in culture. In Vitro 20: 652–662

Moll R, Franke WW, Schiller DL (1982) The catalog of human cytokeratins: patterns of expression in normal epithelia, tumors and cultured cells. Cell 31: 11–24

Moll R, Krepler R, Franke WW (1983) Complex cytokeratin polypeptide patterns observed in certain human carcinomas. Differentiation 23: 256–269

Nagle RG, Boecker W, Davis JR, Heid HW, Kaufmann M, Lucas DO, Jarasch ED (1986) Characterization of breast carcinomas by two monoclonal antibodies distinguishing myoepithelial from luminal epithelial cells. J Histochem Cytochem 34: 869–881

Nishizuka J (1986) Studies and perspectives of protein kinase C. Science 233: 305–312

Osborn M, Franke WW, Weber K (1980) Direct demonstration of the presence of two immunologically distinct intermediate-sized filament systems in the same cell by double immunofluorescence microscopy. Exp Cell Res 125: 37–46

Osborn M, Weber K (1986) Intermediate filament proteins: a multigene family distinguishing major cell lineages. Trends Biochem Sci 11: 469–472

Petersen OW, van Deurs B (1987) Preservation of defined phenotypic traits in short-term cultured human breast carcinoma derived epithelial cells. Cancer Res 47: 856–866

Ramaekers FCS, Haag D, Kant A, Moesker O, Jap PHK, Vooijs GP (1983) Coexpression of keratin- and vimentin-type intermediate filaments in human metastatic carcinoma cells. Proc Nat Acad Sci USA 80: 2618–2622

Rodgers CS, Hill SM, Hulten MA (1984) Cytogenetic analysis in human breast carcinoma. I. Nine cases in the diploid range investigated using direct preparations. Cancer Genet Cytogenet 13: 95–119

Rozengurt E (1986) Early signals in the mitogenic response. Science 234: 161–166

Salomon DS, Perroteau I, Kidwell WR (1986) Tumor-derived growth factors in rodent and human mammary carcinoma cells. Contr Oncol 23: 5–16

Satya-Prakash KL, Pathak S, Hsu TC, Olive M, Cailleau R (1981) Cytogenetic analysis on eight human breast tumor lines. High frequencies of 1q, 11q, and HeLa marker chromosomes. Cancer Genet Cytogenet 3: 61–73

Schor SL, Schor AM (1987) Foetal to adult transitions in fibroblast phenotype: Their possible relevance to the pathogenesis of cancer. J Cell Sci Suppl 8: 165–180

Simon WE, Albrecht M, Trams G, Dietel M, Hölzel F (1984) In vitro growth promotion of human mammary carcinoma cells by steroid hormones, tamoxifen, and prolactin. J Natl Cancer Inst 73: 313–321

Smith HS, Hackett AJ (1987) Use of cells cultured from human mammary carcinomas for studies of malignant progression and chemotherapeutic drug sensitivity. J Lab Clin Med 109: 236–243

Smith HS, Lan S, Ceriani R, Hackett AJ, Stampfer MR (1981) Clonal proliferation of cultured nonmalignant and malignant breast epithelia. Cancer Res 41: 4637–4643

Smith HS, Liotta LA, Hancock MC, Wolman SR, Hackett AJ (1985a) Invasiveness and ploidy of human mammary carcinomas in shortterm cultures. Proc Natl Acad Sci USA 82: 1805–1809

Smith HS, Wolman SR, Auer G, Hackett AJ (1985b) Cell culture studies: a perspective on malignant progression of human breast cancer. In: Rich AM, Hager JC, Taylor-Papadimitriou (eds) Breast cancer: origins, detection, and treatment. Martinus Nijhoff, Boston, pp 75–89

Soule HD, McGrath CM (1986) A simplified method for passage and long-term growth of human mammary epithelial cells. In Vitro Cell Dev Biol 22: 6–12

Stampfer M (1982) Cholera toxin stimulation of human mammary epithelial cells in culture. In Vitro 18: 531–537

Stampfer M, Hallowes RC, Hackett AJ (1980) Growth of normal human mammary cells in culture. In Vitro 16: 415–425

Taylor CM, Blanchard B, Zava DT (1984) A simple method to determine whole cell uptake of radiolabelled oestrogen and progesterone and their subcellular localization in breast cancer cell lines in monolayer culture. J Steroid Biochem 20: 1083–1088

Taylor-Papadimitriou J, Lane BE (1987) Keratin expression in the mammary gland. In: Neville MC, Daniel CW (eds) The mammary gland: development, regulation, and function. Plenum, New York, pp 181–215

Taylor-Papadimitriou J, Purkis P, Fentiman IS (1980) Cholera toxin and analogues of cyclic AMP stimulate the growth of cultured human mammary epithelial cells. J Cell Physiol 102: 317–321

Trent JM (1985) Cytogenetic and molecular biologic alterations in human breast cancer: a review. Breast Cancer Res Treat 5: 221–229

van Netten JP, Algard FT, Coy P, Carlyle SJ, Brigden ML, Thornton KR, Peter S, Fraser T, To MP (1985) Heterogeneous estrogen receptor levels detected via multiple microsamples from individual breast cancers. Cancer 56: 2019–2024

Weber K, Osborn M, Moll R, Wiklund B, Luening B (1984) Tissue polypeptide antigen (TPA) is related to the non-epidermal keratins 8, 18 and 19 typical of simple and non-squamous epithelia: re-evaluation of a human tumor marker. EMBO J 3: 2707–2714

Whitehead RH, Bertoncello I, Webber LM, Pedersen JS (1983) A new human breast carcinoma cell line (PMC 42) with stem cell characteristics. I. Morphologic characterization. J Natl Cancer Inst 70: 649–661

Wolman SR, Smith HS, Stampfer MS, Hackett AJ (1985) Growth of diploid cells from breast cancers. Cancer Genet Cytogenet 16: 49–64

Effects of Steroids and Their Antagonists on Breast Cancer Cells: Therapeutic Implications

P. D. Darbre[1], J. F. Glover[1], and R. J. B. King[2]

[1] Cellular Endocrinology Laboratory, Imperial Cancer Research Fund, Lincoln's Inn Fields, London WC2A 3PX, Great Britain
[2] Hormone Biochemistry Laboratory, Imperial Cancer Research Fund, Lincoln's Inn Fields, London WC2A 3PX, Great Britain

Regulation by Steroids

Steroid hormones regulate the growth of both normal and tumour mammary cells, but the detailed mechanism remains unclear. Regulation is diverse and complex, involving direct effects on the tumour cells and indirect effects via other organs. For this reason, it has been very difficult to interpret data in vivo, and cell culture systems have been extensively used. We use two model systems for study of steroid hormone action in vitro: oestrogen-regulated human mammary tumour cells (ZR-75-I, MCF-7, T-47-D) and androgen-regulated mouse mammary tumour cells (S115).

Questions about steroid hormone regulation of cultured breast tumour cells can essentially be broken down into two parts. Firstly, one can ask in the short-term, how do steroid hormones control tumour cell growth? Whilst a major issue here is obviously of steroid effects on the rate of cell proliferation, regulation of other cell biological parameters such as density regulation, cell morphology and growth in suspension are pertinent to the growth of tumour cells. Secondly, the longer-term question asks why breast cancer cells progress from a state of steroid sensitivity to one of steroid insensitivity. This is of major clinical importance since in humans only 30% of breast cancers regress under endocrine therapy. Even then, this regression is often temporary and replaced by growth of hormone-independent tumours. We discuss here studies of cultured breast cancer cells which have aided us in our understanding of the mechanism of steroid hormone action.

Short-term Effects

Early events in steroid action involve the binding of steroid to its specific receptor within the cell (King 1987) and molecular studies have now defined regions in the DNA which bind the hormone-receptor complexes (Ponta et al. 1985). However, later events remain within an unknown "black box". We have attempted to define specific post-receptor events which are regulated by steroids at both a cellular and molecular level.

At a cellular level, growth has been studied as either anchorage-dependent (monolayer culture) or anchorage-independent (suspension culture), and each can be described in terms of log-phase proliferation rate, saturation density or cell morphology. Oestradiol alters all these parameters for human breast cancer cell lines (Figs. 1, 2). Steroid-regulated changes in cell morphology are documented in the literature (Sapino et al. 1986; Vic et al. 1982). We have previously argued that the proliferation seen in the absence of added oestrogen was not due to residual oestrogen in the serum (Darbre et al. 1983a). Recently, it has been shown that the pH indicator, phenol red, found in all tissue culture media can act as a weak oestrogen (Berthois et al. 1986). In the absence of phenol red, ZR-75-I cells exhibit less proliferation in the absence of oestradiol (Fig. 3). It is clear from now on that any studies of oestrogenic or antioestrogenic effects on cells in culture must be performed in the absence of phenol red.

Our other model system has involved use of the cloned S115 mouse mammary tumour cells which are responsive to both androgen and glucocorticoid (Darbre

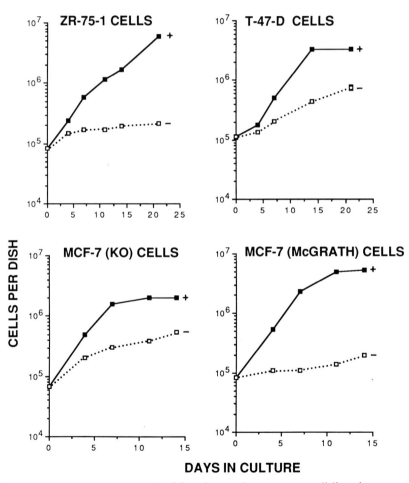

Fig. 1. Effects of estradiol on the growth of four human breast cancer cell lines in monolayer culture. Cells were grown in the absence of phenol red with $(+)$ ($\blacksquare$——$\blacksquare$) or without $(-)$ ($\square$----$\square$) $10^{-8} M$ oestradiol

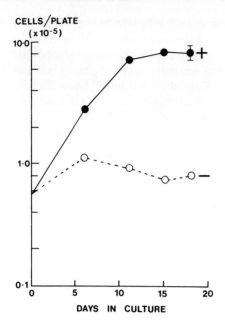

CELLS/PLATE
(x 10⁻⁵)

DAYS IN CULTURE

Fig. 2. Effects of oestradiol on the growth of human breast cancer cells ZR-75-I in suspension culture. Cells were grown in the absence of phenol red with $(+)$ ($\bullet$——$\bullet$) or without $(-)$ ($\circ$----$\circ$) $10^{-8}M$ oestradiol

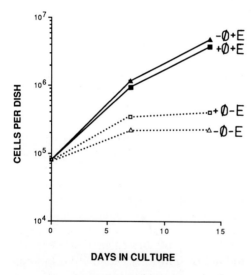

CELLS PER DISH

DAYS IN CULTURE

Fig. 3. Effects of phenol red on the growth of human breast cancer cells ZR-75-I in monolayer culture. Cells were grown with or without 15 mg/litre phenol red (φ), with or without $10^{-8}M$ oestradiol *(E)*

and King 1987a). Both steroids increase saturation density in monolayer and growth in suspension (Fig. 4), and both cause a marked changed from epithelial morphology (without hormone) to fibroblastic morphology (with hormone) (Couchman et al. 1981). However, they have opposing effects on log-phase proliferation rate (Fig. 4). This serves to emphasise that different steroids do not necessarily have the same effects on each cell biological parameter (Darbre et al. 1987a).

From these studies, we have developed the model that in cell biological terms, androgens convert S115 cells from a normal ($-$hormone) to a transformed ($+$hor-

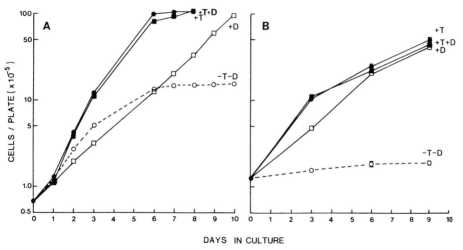

Fig. 4 A, B. Effects of androgen and glucocorticoid on growth of S115 mouse mammary tumour cells in **A** monolayer or **B** suspension culture. Cells were grown with or without $3.5 \times 10^{-8} M$ testosterone *(T)*, with or without $10^{-7} M$ dexamethasone *(D)*

mone) phenotype (Couchman et al. 1981; Yates et al. 1980). Since these cells are tumour cells, such alterations cannot be linked directly to tumorigenesis in vivo, but they do indicate some fundamental effects of steroids. In view of the well-documented involvement of mouse mammary tumour virus (MMTV) in the development of mammary carcinomas in the mouse (Michalides et al. 1983), we wondered if viral elements could be involved in these steroid-regulated changes in the S115 cell line. No viral particles have been detected, but S115 cells possess both endogenous MMTV proviral units in DNA and RNAs transcribed from them, which are regulated by androgen and glucocorticoid (Darbre et al. 1983b, 1985). The physiological function of these RNAs has still to be established, but at the very least, they provide both a useful early marker of postreceptor events and information about steroid regulation of MMTV. It is well established that MMTV RNA production is regulated by glucocorticoids through a proviral long terminal repeat (LTR) sequence (Ringold 1983). However, the regulation of MMTV RNA by both androgen and glucocorticoid in S115 cells raised the possibility of multi-hormonal regulation on the LTR. In fact, it is now evident that the LTR can be regulated directly, not only by glucocorticoid, but also by androgens (Darbre et al. 1986), progesterone (Cato et al. 1986), and aldosterone (Cato et al. 1987) but not by oestrogen. Such regulation brings new biological relevance to steroid regulation of MMTV in breast cancer. Since regulatory elements in DNA for different steroid hormones share some structural similarities (von der Ahe et al. 1985), it is perhaps not surprising to find multi-hormonal regulation of certain genes, and indeed it appears from these simple transfection experiments that there are two types of steroid for gene regulation: class I glucocorticoid/androgen/progesterone/aldosterone and class II oestrogen. Evidently, such regulation does not simply follow receptor status of the cells nor is it necessarily reflected in growth regulation by the steroids (Table 1).

Table 1. Steroid regulation of gene expression: Correlation of steroid regulation of transfected LTR sequences with receptor status and steroid effects on cell proliferation

Cells	Steroid receptors	Regulation of transfected LTR	Effects on cell proliferation
S115	T D	T D	T↑D↓
T47D	E P T D	P T D	E↑ P↓ T↓ D↑

D, dexamethasone; *E,* oestradiol; *P,* progesterone; *T,* testosterone; ↑, growth increased; ↓, growth decreased.

Loss of Response

Manipulation of the steroid environment affects breast tumour growth in many species, and endocrine therapy of breast cancer has been developed on this basis. However, only some breast tumours respond to such therapy, and of those, regression is often temporary and is replaced by unresponsive tumours. A recent approach to breast cancer management has been to select hormone-sensitive tumours by measuring their oestrogen and progesterone receptor levels (DeSombre and Jensen 1982). Implicit in this is the assumption that loss of receptor is a fundamental cause of steroid insensitivity, but is it?

It is now accepted that the origin of mammary tumours is monoclonal, but tumours themselves are composed of very mixed populations of cells. Steroid sensitivity/insensitivity is just one of many phenotypes which diverge during tumour progression. Such diversity could arise by either a genotypic or phenotypic mechanism. Evidence for the former is well-established (Kim 1985), but evidence that phenotypic mechanisms may be involved in loss of steroid sensitivity is now emerging and is encouraging in terms of therapeutic possibilities (Darbre and King 1985; Nicholson 1985).

Experiments designed to elucidate the origin of such heterogeneity are fraught with difficulties, and the best way in which meaningful data can be obtained is to study the divergence of cloned cells in tissue culture. We started our studies using cloned S115 cells as an in vitro model and are now moving to using cloned human cells also. Such analyses involve long-term growth of these cells in tissue culture in the absence of steroid, together with analyses of steroid sensitive parameters at regular intervals.

Prolonged withdrawal of steroid from cloned S115 mouse mammary tumour cells results in a rapid, ordered, reproducible series of phenotypic changes culminating in loss of both cellular and molecular steroid-sensitive parameters (Darbre and King 1984) (see Table 2). Thus, a clone of responsive cells can give rise reproducibly to a population of unresponsive cells solely upon removal of steroid. The time course of loss of steroid sensitivity has been determined in terms of loss of proliferative, saturation density and morphological responses in monolayer (Darbre and King 1984), in terms of responses in suspension growth (Darbre and King 1987a) and in terms of loss of MMTV RNA (Darbre and King 1984). Initial changes were reversible, but later changes became irreversible. At the stage when MMTV RNA was irreversibly lost, an increased methylation of MMTV-LTR se-

Table 2. Characteristics of steroid-responsive ($+$A) and steroid-unresponsive ($-$A) S115 mouse mammary tumour cells

Property	$+$A Cells		$-$A Cells	
	$+$T	$+$G	$+$T	$+$G
1. Monolayer growth				
Proliferative response	Yes ↑	Yes ↓	No	No
Morphological response	Yes ↑	Yes ↑	No	No
Saturation density response	Yes ↑	Yes ↑	No	No
Cell morphology	F ⇌ E		Elongated epithelial	
2. Suspension growth				
Proliferative response	Yes ↑	Yes ↑	No	No
Maximal density response	Yes ↑	Yes ↑	No	No
Colony morphology	Tightly clustered spheroids		Loosely clustered spheroids	
3. MMTV RNA	Yes	Yes	No	No
Molecular response	Yes ↑	Yes ↑	No	No
4. Receptors	Yes	Yes	Yes	Yes

$+$ T, with testosterone; $+$ G, with glucocorticoid; F, fibroblastic morphology (with T or G); E, epithelial morphology (without any hormone); ↑, increased response; ↓, decreased response.

quences in the DNA was detected (Darbre and King 1987b). Since this DNA methylation occurs many weeks after the RNA has been lost, it cannot be responsible for the initial loss of the RNA, but it is possible that it could be involved in the final irreversible steps towards steroid insensitivity.

Normal and tumour mammary cells have complex endocrine requirements, yet most studies of the origin of steroid-insensitive cells have concentrated on the loss of response to only one steroid. Since the S115 cells are responsive to both androgen and glucocorticoid, we have recently had the opportunity of studying the interaction of two steroids during progression to steroid autonomy. Interestingly, the cells could be protected against any loss of response to either androgen or glucocorticoid with either steroid alone. Androgen protects against loss of glucocorticoid sensitivity, and glucocorticoid protects against loss of androgen sensitivity (Darbre and King 1987b).

The majority of steroid hormone effects are mediated by intracellular receptor proteins. However, the transition from the steroid-sensitive to the -insensitive state is not always associated with loss of receptor. Examples of receptor-positive but steroid-insensitive cells have been described (Daniel et al. 1986; Darbre and King 1987c; Gaubert et al. 1986; Gehring 1986; George and Wilson 1986; King 1978; Kontula et al. 1986; Miesfeld et al. 1984; Nawata et al. 1981; Sedlacek and Horwitz 1984; Sibley and Yamamoto 1979; Westphal et al. 1984). In some cases, the ineffectiveness of the steroid receptor complex is due to abnormal receptors with defects distal to the initial steroid binding step (Danielson et al. 1986; Miesfeld et al. 1984; Westphal et al. 1984), but sometimes the receptors are normal (Darbre and King 1987c; Gaubert et al. 1986; King 1978; Sibley and Yamamoto 1979). The loss of hormone-sensitive parameters in the S115 cells also occurs without either loss of receptor number (King 1978) or of receptor function (Darbre and King 1987c). Receptor number was measured by a steroid binding assay, but receptor function was assessed using transfection as a biological assay.

Loss of steroid sensitivity is a feature also of the human breast cancer cell lines grown in the absence of steroid. This ist true for the cloned MCF-7 line (Katzenellenbogen et al. 1987), ZR-75-I cell line (Fig. 5) and T-47-D cell line (Fig. 6). As for the mouse cells, steroid deprivation results in a slow phase of growth followed by increased growth. Interestingly, growth in the absence of steroid (and phenol red) is abolished after 3 weeks for ZR-75-I cells but not for T-47-D cells, suggesting that there exist both cells which are dependent (ZR-75-I) and responsive

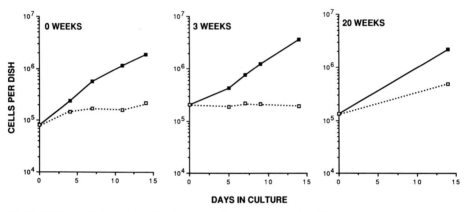

Fig. 5. Effects of steroid deprivation on subsequent growth of human breast cancer cells ZR-75-I in monolayer culture. Cells were grown initially for 0, 3 or 20 weeks without steroid or phenol red. Then growth was assessed in the absence of phenol red with ($\blacksquare$——$\blacksquare$) or without ($\square$----$\square$) $10^{-8} M$ oestradiol

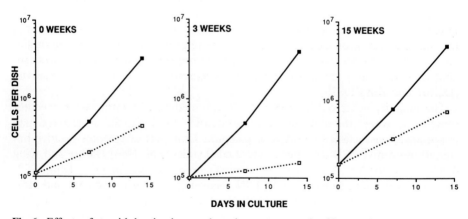

Fig. 6. Effects of steroid deprivation on the subsequent growth of human breast cancer cells T-47-D in monolayer culture. Cells were grown initially for 0, 3 or 15 weeks without steroid or phenol red. Then growth was assessed in the absence of phenol red with ($\blacksquare$——$\blacksquare$) or without ($\square$----$\square$) $10^{-8} M$ oestradiol

(T-47-D) on oestradiol for growth. Longer-term steroid deprivation results in re-sumed growth in both cell lines. However, unlike for the mouse cells, readdition of steroid at any stage resulted in immediate resumption of normal growth. In the case of the MCF-7 cells, these changes occurred in the face of normal induction of progesterone receptor by oestradiol (Katzenellenbogen et al. 1987), indicating that as for the mouse cells such changes do not involve any loss of receptor func-tion.

Effects of Steroid Antagonists

The theoretical definition of a steroid antagonist is a compound that inhibits the effect of a steroid, but in practice they can also have effects in their own right (Knabbe et al. 1987; Vignon et al. 1987). In terms of breast cancer, the main con-siderations here are of anti-oestrogens, such as tamoxifen and trans-hydroxy-tamoxifen, which have become clinically important in endocrine therapy of breast cancer (Jordan 1986).

Effects on Growth

The use of tissue-cultured cells to test the effects of anti-oestrogens provides a very powerful model system, but most studies to date have utilised culture media con-taining phenol red, implying that they have all been done against a background of low oestrogen. Such studies revealed that tamoxifen stimulated cell growth in a dose-dependent manner up to $10^{-7}M$, but inhibition was observed at $10^{-6}M$ (Dar-bre et al. 1984; Reddel and Sutherland 1984). Consistent anti-oestrogenic effects of tamoxifen required an oestradiol: tamoxifen ratio of 1:1000 (Darbre et al. 1984).

It now appears that tamoxifen and trans-hydroxytamoxifen act on MCF-7 cells in tissue culture only by antagonising phenol red-stimulated proliferation and have no effect in the absence of phenol red (Berthois et al. 1986). We have recently re-examined the effects of these compounds on the growth of ZR-75-I cells in the absence of phenol red (Fig. 7). At high cell density, tamoxifen gave weak stimula-tory effects whilst trans-hydroxy-tamoxifen showed no significant action. How-ever, at low cell density, the story was different. Tamoxifen showed a biphasic ac-tion: initial weak stimulation followed by later inhibition. Trans-hydroxytamox-ifen did not stimulate, but inhibition increased with time in culture. In these exper-iments, we were struck by the observation that tamoxifen only inhibited the cells at later times when growth in the absence of steroid had stopped (Fig. 7). Further experiments showed that after 3 weeks' deprivation of steroid, when growth of the cells had ceased (Fig. 5), anti-oestrogen action became only inhibitory at low den-sity (Fig. 8). We have thus concluded that anti-oestrogen action in vitro is affected by at least four parameters; (a) presence of phenol red, (b) time in culture, (c) cell density, and (d) levels of basal cell growth. The cell density effects could be due to differential anti-oestrogen action on exponentially growing and plateau phase

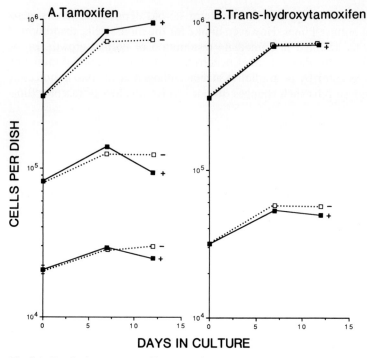

Fig. 7 A, B. Anti-oestrogen effects on the growth of human breast cancer cells ZR-75-I in monolayer culture at different cell densities. Cells were grown without oestradiol and in the absence of phenol red: **A** with (■——■) or without (□----□) $10^{-6}M$ tamoxifen; **B** with (■——■) or without (□----□) $10^{-8}M$ trans-hydroxytamoxifen

cells (Sutherland et al. 1983) or alternatively to varying levels of autocrine growth-stimulating factors (Vignon et al. 1987).

Scientific Conclusions

1. Steroids regulate the growth of breast cancer cells, and cells exist which are both responsive to and dependent on steroids for proliferation. Steroids affect many cell biological parameters, and different steroids can have differential effects.
2. Molecular markers of steroid action have been defined in S115 mouse mammary tumour cells and multi-hormonal regulation of genes established.
3. A clone of responsive cells can give rise to a population of unresponsive cells solely by removal of hormone. Such loss of response is reversible initially but ultimately becomes irreversible. DNA methylation could play a role in irreversible events.
4. Several hormones can interact in loss of steroid sensitivity.
5. Loss of steroid sensitivity can occur in the face of fully functional receptors.
6. Anti-oestrogens antagonize oestrogen-regulated growth of cultured cells but on their own have different effects determined by at least four parameters: (a) presence of phenol red, (b) time in culture, (c) cell density and (d) basal cell growth.

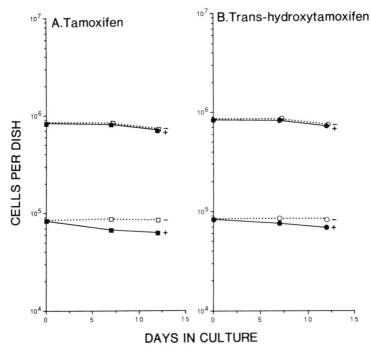

Fig. 8 A, B. Anti-oestrogen effects on the growth of steroid-deprived human breast cancer cells ZR-75-I in monolayer culture at different cell densities. Cells were grown firstly for 3 weeks without steroid in the absence of phenol red. Then growth was assessed in the absence of estradiol or phenol red but **A** with ($\blacksquare\!-\!\blacksquare$) or without ($\square\text{-----}\square$) $10^{-6} M$ tamoxifen; **B** with ($\blacksquare\!-\!\blacksquare$) or without ($\square\text{-----}\square$) $10^{-8} M$ trans-hydroxytamoxifen

Therapeutic Implications

1. Cell biology studies emphasise the need to antagonize not only the proliferative effects of steroids but also other growth parameters.
2. A phenotypic mechanism in loss of response implies that events may be both reversible and preventable. Since it occurs purely by removal of steroid in culture, regimes of steroid ablation may not be the best form of long-term therapy and may actually accelerate the production of unresponsive cells.
3. Involvement of DNA methylation in loss of response suggests that treatment with drugs such as azacytidine might be worth considering.
4. Interaction of steroids during loss of response should be considered in design of therapy. The identification of one receptor type in a tumour may increase the probability of response to other steroids. Indeed, oestrogen receptor assays do have predictive value for response to all types of endocrine therapy.
5. Since complete insensitivity can be generated in the face of a fully functional receptor machinery, this explains the existence of the breast tumours which possess steroid receptors yet which do not respond to endocrine therapy. This implies that receptor assays alone will never predict response perfectly. Receptor-

negative tumours will not respond to therapy, but the presence of receptor alone cannot guarantee response.
6. Studies of anti-oestrogen action suggest that such compounds do antagonize oestrogen action but also have effects in their own right. The cell density effects suggest that these agents may be more effective in vivo on tumours of low cellularity and that areas within a tumour packed densely with malignant cells may be difficult to attack with anti-oestrogens alone. The biphasic action to tamoxifen in culture may explain the response in vivo of tamoxifen tumour flare where there is an early rise in tumour size before regression.

References

Berthois Y, Katzenellenbogen JA, Katzenellenbogen BS (1986) Phenol red in tissue culture media is a weak estrogen: Implications concerning the study of estrogen-responsive cells in culture. Proc Natl Acad Sci USA 83: 2496–2500

Cato ACB, Miksicek R, Schutz G, Arnemann J, Beato M (1986) The hormone regulatory element of mouse mammary tumour virus mediates progesterone induction. EMBO J 5: 2237–2240

Cato ACB, Skroch P, Butkeraitis P, Ponat H (1988) The multi-hormonal regulation of transcription at the mouse mammary tumour virus promoter. In: Bresciani F, King RJB, Lippman ME, Raynaud JP (eds) Hormones and cancer, vol 3. Raven, New York, pp 114–117 (Progress in cancer research and therapy, vol 35)

Couchman JR, Yates J, King RJB, Badley RA (1981) Changes in microfilament and focal adhesion distribution with loss of androgen responsiveness in cultured mammary tumor cells. Cancer Res 41: 263–269

Danielson M, Northrop JP, Ringold GM (1986) The mouse glucocorticoid receptor: Mapping of functional domains by cloning, sequencing and expression of wild-type and mutant receptor proteins. EMBO J 5: 2513–2522

Darbre P, King RJB (1984) Progression to steroid autonomy in SII5 mouse mammary tumor cells: Role of DNA methylation. J Cell Biol 99: 1410–1415

Darbre PD, King RJB (1987a) Differential effects of steroid hormones on parameters of cell growth. Cancer Res 47: 2937–2944

Darbre PD, King RJB (1987b) Interaction of different steroid hormones during progression of tumour cells to steroid autonomy. Int J Cancer 40: 802–806

Darbre PD, King RJB (1987c) Progression to steroid insensitivity can occur irrespective of the presence of functional steroid receptors. Cell 51: 521–528

Darbre P, Yates J, Curtis S, King RJB (1983a) Effect of estradiol on human breast cancer cells in culture. Cancer Res 43: 349–354

Darbre P, Dickson C, Petes G, Page M, Curtis S, King RJB (1983b) Androgen regulation of cell proliferation and expression of viral sequences in mouse mammary tumour cells. Nature 303: 431–433

Darbre PD, Curtis S, King RJB (1984) Effects of estradiol and tamoxifen on human breast cancer cells in serum-free culture. Cancer Res 44: 2790–2793

Darbre PD, Moriarty A, Curtis SA, King RJB (1985) Androgen regulates MMTV RNA in the short term in SII5 mouse mammary tumour cells. J Steroid Biochem 23: 379–384

Darbre P, Page M, King RJB (1986) Androgen regulation by the long terminal repeat of mouse mammary tumor virus. Mol Cell Biol 6: 2847–2854

DeSombre ER, Jensen EV (1982) Clinical usefulness of steroid receptor determinations in breast cancer. In: Leung BS (ed) Hormonal regulation of mammary tumors, vol 1. Eden, Montreal, Canada, pp 155–182

Gaubert CM, Carriero R, Shyamala G (1986) Relationships between mammary estrogen receptor and estrogenic sensitivity: Molecular properties of cytoplasmic receptor and its binding to deoxyribonucleic acid. Endocrinology 118: 1504–1512

Gehring U (1986) Genetics of glucocorticoid receptors. Mol Cel Endocrinol 48: 89–96

George FW, Wilson JD (1986) Hormonal control of sexual development. Vitam Horm 43: 145–196

Jordan VC (ed) (1986) Estrogen/antiestrogen action and breast cancer therapy. University of Wisconsin Press, Madison, Wisconsin

Katzenellenbogen BS, Kendra KL, Norman MJ, Berthois Y (1987) Proliferation, hormonal responsiveness and estrogen receptor content of MCF-7 human breast cancer cells grown in the short-term and long-term absence of estrogens. Cancer Res 47: 4355–4360

Kim U (1985) Factors influencing the generation of phenotypic herterogeneity in mammary tumors. In: Mihich E (ed) Biological responses in cancer, vol 4. Plenum, New York, pp 91–124

King RJB (1978) Studies on the regulation of cell proliferation in culture by steroids. In: Dumont J, Nunez J (eds) Hormones and cell regulation, vol 2. Elsevier-North Holland Biomedical, Amsterdam, pp 15–36

King RJB (1987) Structure and function of steroid receptors. J Endocrinol 114: 341–349

Knabbe C, Lippman ME, Wakefield LM, Flanders KC, Kasid A, Derynck R, Dickson RB (1987) Evidence that transforming growth factor-β is a hormonally regulated negative growth factor in human breast cancer cells. Cell 48: 417–428

Kontula KK, Janne OA, Bardin CW (1986) Intracellular hormone receptor defects and disease. In: Conn PM (ed) The receptors, vol 4. Academic, New York, pp 37–74

Michalides R, van Ooyen A, Nusse R (1983) Mouse mammary tumor virus expression and mammary tumor development. Curr Top Microbiol Immunol 106: 57–78

Miesfeld R, Okret S, Wikstrom AC, Wrange O, Gustafsson JA, Yamamoto KR (1984) Characterization of a steroid hormone receptor gene and mRNA in wild-type and mutant cells. Nature 312: 779–781

Nawata H, Chong MT, Bronzert D, Lippman ME (1981) Estrogen-independent growth of a subline of MCF-7 human breast cancer cells in culture. J Biol Chem 256: 6895–6902

Nicholson GL (1985) The evolution of phenotypic diversity in metastatic tumor cells. In: Mihich E (ed) Biological responses in cancer, vol 4. Plenum New York, pp 71–89

Ponta H, Günzberg WH, Salmons B, Groner B, Herrlich P (1985) Mouse mammary tumour virus: A proviral gene contributes to the understanding of eukaryotic gene expression and mammary tumorigenesis. J Gen Virol 66: 931–943

Reddel RR, Sutherland RL (1984) Tamoxifen stimulation of human breast cancer cell proliferation in vitro. A possible model for tamoxifen tumour flare. Eur J Cancer Clin Oncol 20: 1419–1424

Ringold GM (1983) Regulation of mouse mammary tumor virus gene expression by glucocorticoid hormones. Curr Top Microbiol Immunol 106: 79–103

Sapino A, Pietribiasi F, Bussolati G, Marchisio PC (1986) Estrogen- and tamoxifen-induced rearrangement of cytoskeleton and adhesion structures in breast cancer MCF-7 cells. Cancer Res 46: 2526–2531

Sedlacek SM, Horwitz KB (1984) The role of progestins and progesterone receptors in the treatment of breast cancer. Steroids 44: 467–484

Sibley CH, Yamamoto KR (1979) Mouse lymphoma cells: Mechanisms of resistance to glucocorticoids. In: Baxter JD, Rousseau GG (eds) Glucocorticoid hormone action. Springer, New York Berlin Heidelberg, pp 357–376 (Monographs in endocrinology, vol 12)

Sutherland RL, Hall RE, Taylor IW (1983) Cell proliferation kinetics of MCF-7 human mammary carcinoma cells in culture and effects of tamoxifen on exponentially growing and plateau-phase cells. Cancer Res 43: 3988–4006

Vic P, Vignon F, Deroc D, Rochefort H (1982) Effect of estradiol on the ultrastructure of the MCF-7 human breast cancer cells in culture. Cancer Res 42: 667–673

Vignon F, Bouton MM, Rochefort M (1987) Antiestrogens inhibit the mitogenic effect of growth factors on breast cancer cells in the total absence of estrogens. Biochem Biophs Res Commun 146: 1502–1508

von der Ahe D, Janich S, Scheidereit C, Renkawitz R, Schutz G, Beato M (1985) Glucocorticoid and progesterone receptors bind to the same sites in two hormonally regulated promoters. Nature 313: 706–709

Westphal HM, Mugele K, Beato M, Gehring U (1984) Immunochemical characterization of wild-type and variant glucocorticoid receptors by monoclonal antibodies EMBO J 3: 1493–1498

Yates J, Couchman JR, King RJB (1980) Androgen effects on growth, morphology, and sensitivity of SIIS mouse mammary tumour cells in culture. In: King RJG, Iacobelli S, Lindner HR, Lippman ME (eds) Hormones and cancer, vol 14. Raven, New York, pp 31–39

Estrogen-Induced Mitogens in Breast Cancer and Their Prognostic Value

F. Vignon, P. Briozzo, F. Capony, M. Garcia, G. Freiss, M. Morisset, and H. Rochefort

Unité Hormones et Cancer (U 148), INSERM, 60, rue de Navacelles, 34090 Montpellier, France

The establishment of numerous breast cancer cell lines in continuous culture has favored the study of the hormonal control of breast cancer proliferation in the past years.

In hormone-responsive breast cancer cells (estrogen-receptor positive) estrogens were shown to modulate rapidly the expression of various proteins and peptides and finally to stimulate their proliferation (Adams et al. 1983; Rochefort et al. 1984; Lippman et al. 1986). The rapid induction of some secreted proteins has attracted interest in the possibility of an estrogen-induced autocrine loop of breast cancer growth regulation (Rochefort et al. 1980). It was in fact shown that serum-free conditioned media from estrogen-treated cells did contain autocrine mitogens, thus demonstrating that some estrogen-induced proteins and peptides could serve as mediators of estrogen action on cell growth (Vignon et al. 1983; Lippman et al. 1986).

With the aim of identifying such autocrine mitogens, we have focussed our study on a 52000-dalton glycoprotein which is induced by estradiol and secreted by breast cancer cells (Westley and Rochefort 1980). Several high-affinity monoclonal antibodies have allowed the purification of the secretory 52K protein to homogeneity (Garcia et al. 1985; Capony et al. 1986) and to detect its cellular presence under different processed forms (Morisset et al. 1986a). The 52K protein has been identified by biochemical (Capony et al. 1986) and molecular biological means (Augereau et al. 1988) as the secreted precursor of a protease, namely cathepsin D, bearing mannose-6-phosphate signals and routed to lysosomes via mannose-6-phosphate receptor (von Figura and Hasilik 1986).

The purified 52K-cathepsin D was shown to be mitogenic for steroid-deprived breast cancer cells, thus indicating that it is one potential estrogen-induced autocrine mitogen, although the mechanisms by which it regulates cell proliferation remain unclear (Vignon et al. 1986). However, the simultaneous production by breast cancer cells of several peptides identical or analogous to the growth factors (IGF1, IGF2, TGF$_\alpha$, FGF, PDGF ...) (Lippman et al. 1986) suggests a possible indirect stimulatory pathway via its proteolytic activity through activation of the growth factor precursor or inactive latent form (Derynck et al. 1984; Gospodarowicz et al. 1986). Moreover, the recent identification of the high homology between the mannose-6-phosphate receptor and the IGF2 receptor suggests that this protease could directly stimulate mitogenesis (Morgan et al. 1987) via its interaction with this receptor.

Recent Results in Cancer Research, Vol. 113
© Springer-Verlag Berlin·Heidelberg 1989

The 52K-cathepsin D is also able to degrade specific substrate (Morisset et al. 1986b), basement membrane and proteoglycans (Capony et al. 1987), following its activation at acidic pH. This ability to digest extracellular matrix in vitro (Briozzo et al. 1988) associated to the evidence that the protease is secreted in larger amounts by cancer cells than by normal cells (Capony et al., to be published) have suggested that it might be implicated in breast cancer invasion and metastatic processes.

Clinical retrospective studies in collaboration with Rose and Thorpe (Copenhagen) on a series of 154 postmenopausal patients with 6 years follow-up support this assumption. Immunoenzymatic assays of the 52K-cathepsin D concentrations in primary tumor cytosols have shown that a high concentration of protease is an independent prognosis factor associated with a shorter disease-free survival (Thorpe et al. to be published).

The estrogen-induced 52K-cathepsin D is also constitutively produced by estrogen receptor-negative breast cancer cells and appears to be more related to cell proliferation than to hormone dependency (Garcia et al. 1987). Immunohistochemical studies have additionally indicated that it is elevated in high-risk mastopathies (Garcia et al. 1986).

In conclusion, 52K-cathepsin D may have important autocrine and paracrine functions in stimulating the growth and invasion of hormone-responsive and -unresponsive breast cancers and appears to be a useful tissue marker to predict high-risk mastopathies and breast cancer invasiveness (Rochefort et al. 1987).

References

Adams DJ, Edwards DP, McGuire WL (1983) Estrogen regulation of specific proteins as a mode of hormone action in human breast cancer. Biomembranes 11: 389

Augereau P, Garcia M, Mattei MG, Cavaillès V, Depadova F, Derocq D, Capony F, Ferrara P, Rochefort H (1988) Cloning and sequencing of the 52K cathepsin D eDNA of MCF7 breast cancer cells and mapping on chromosome II. Mol Endocrinol 2: 186

Briozzo P, Morisset M, Capony F, Rougeot C, Rochefort H (1988) In vitro degradation of extracellular matrix with 52K cathepsin D secreted by breast cancer cells. Cancer Res 48: 3688

Capony F, Garcia M, Capdevielle J, Rougeot C, Ferrara P, Rochefort H (1986) Purification and characterization of the secreted and cellular 52-kDa proteins regulated by estrogens in human breast cancer cells. Eur J Biochem 161: 505

Capony F, Morisset M, Barrett AJ, Capony JM, Broquet P, Vignon F, Chambon M, Louisot P, Rochefort H (1987) Phosphorylation, glycosylation and proteolytic activity of the 52K estrogen-induced protein secreted by MCF7 cells. J Cell Biol 104: 253

Derynck R, Roberts AB, Winkler ME, Chen EY, Goeddel DV (1984) Human transforming growth factor: Precursor structure and expression in E.Coli. Cell 38: 287

Dickson RB, McManaway ME, Lippman ME (1986) Estrogen-induced factors of breast cancer cells partially replace estrogen to promote tumor growth. Science 232: 1540

Garcia M, Capony F, Derocq D, Simon D, Pau B, Rochefort H (1985) Monoclonal antibodies to the estrogen-regulated Mr 52000 glycoprotein: Characterization and immunodetection in MCF7 cells. Cancer Res 45: 709

Garcia M, Salazar-Retana G, Pages A, Richer G, Domergue J, Pages AM, Cavalié G, Martin JM, Lamarque JL, Pau B, Pujol H, Rochefort H (1986) Distribution of the Mr 52000 estrogen-regulated protein in benign breast diseases and other tissues by immunohistochemistry. Cancer Res 46: 3734

Garcia M, Contesso G, Duplay H, Cavaillès V, Derocq D, Delarue JC, Krebs B, Sancho-Garnier H, Richer G, Domergue J, Namer M, Rochefort H (1987) Immunohistochemical distribution of the 52K protein in mammary tumors: A marker associated to cell proliferation rather than to hormone responsiveness. J Steroid Biochem 27: 439

Gospodarowicz D, Neufeld G, Schweigerer L (1986) Fibroblast growth factor. Mol Cell Endocrinol 46: 187

Lippman ME, Dickson RB, Bates S, Knabbe C, Huff K, Swain S, McManaway M, Bronzert D, Kasid A, Gelmann EP (1986) Autocrine and paracrine growth regulation of human breast cancer. Breast Cancer Res Treat 1: 59

Morgan DO, Edman JC, Standring DN, Fried VA, Smith MC, Roth RA, Rutter WJ (1987) Insulin like growth factor II receptor as a multifunctional binding protein. Nature 329: 301

Morisset M, Capony F, Rochefort H (1986a) Processing and estrogen regulation of the 52-kDa protein inside MCF7 breast cancer cells. Endocrinology 119: 2773

Morisset M, Capony F, Rochefort H (1986b) The 52-kDa estrogen induced protein secreted by MCF7 cells is a lysosomal acidic protease. Biochem Biophys Res Commun 138: 505

Rochefort H, Coezy E, Joly E, Westley B, Vignon F (1980) Hormonal control of breast cancer in cell culture. In: Iacobelli S, King R, Lindner H, Lippman M (eds) Hormones and cancer. Raven, New York, pp 21 (Progress in cancer research and therapy, vol 14)

Rochefort H, Chalbos D, Capony F, Garcia M, Veith F, Vignon F, Westley B (1984) Effect of estrogen in breast cancer cells in culture: released proteins and control of cell proliferation. In: Gurpide E, Calandra R, Levy C, Soto RJ (eds) Hormones and cancer, vol 142. Liss, New York, p 37

Rochefort H, Capony F, Garcia M, Cavaillès V, Freiss G, Chambon M, Morisset M, Vignon F (1987) Estrogen-induced lysosomal proteases secreted by breast cancer cells: A role in carcinogenesis? J Cell Biochem 35: 17

Thorpe SM, Rochefort H, Garcia M, Freiss G, Christensen IJ, Khalaf S, Paolucci F, Pau B, Rasmussen BB, Rose C. High concentrations of 52K cathepsin-D predict poor prognosis in primary, postmenopausal breast cancer (submitted for publication)

Vignon F, Derocq D, Chambon M, Rochefort H (1983) Endocrinologie. Les protéines oestrogéno-induites sécrétées par les cellules mammaires cancéreuses humaines MCF7 stimulent leur prolifération. CR Seances Acad Sci 296: 151

Vignon F, Capony F, Chambon M, Freiss G, Garcia M, Rochefort H (1986) Autocrine growth stimulation of the MCF 7 breast cancer cells by the estrogen-regulated 52K protein. Endocrinology 118: 1537

Von Figura K, Hasilik A (1985) Lysosomal enzymes and their receptors. Ann Rev Biochem 55: 167

Westley B, Rochefort H (1980) A secreted glycoprotein induced by estrogen in human breast cancer cell lines. Cell 20: 352

Serum Tyrosine Kinase Activity and Neoplastic Disease

P. L. Lee and G. M. Clinton

Howard Hughes Medical Institute, University of California, School of Medicine, Box 0724, San Francisco, CA 94143, USA

Introduction

Evidence is accumulating that links proto-oncogenes to the induction or maintenance of human malignancies. Much of the evidence is derived from studies of animal models (Bishop 1983) and analyses of proto-oncogenes and their expression in human tumor cell lines and human tumors (Brodeur et al. 1984; Xu et al. 1984).

Many of the proto-oncogenes encode proteins that have tyrosine protein kinase activity (Hunter and Cooper 1985). The proto-oncogene products of the tyrosine kinase family can be divided into two groups. One group includes the growth factor receptors which are transmembrane glycoproteins that promote growth by binding to specific growth factors or by alterations in the regulatory regions of the proteins (Yarden et al. 1986). Contained in this group is the receptor for the macrophage colony-stimulating factor (CSF) which is highly homologous to the transforming gene of the feline sarcoma virus (Sherr et al. 1985), the receptor for epidermal growth factor (EGF) which is homologous to the transforming gene of the avian erythroblastosis virus (Downward et al. 1984), and the protein encoded by the HER-2 protooncogene, the structure of which indicates that it is also likely to be a cellular receptor for an unknown ligand (Padht et al. 1982; Schechter et al. 1984). The second group is typified by the c-src protein which is homologous to the transforming gene product of Rous sarcoma virus. The members of this group are cytoplasmic proteins that neither span the plasma membrane nor are known to be regulated by extracellular ligands (Bishop 1983; Hunter and Cooper 1985).

In most cases, when a member of the tyrosine kinase family promotes cell growth and malignant transformation, there is an amplification in the enzyme activity resulting in the unscheduled tyrosine phosphorylation of cellular proteins (Hunter and Cooper 1985). Tyrosine kinase activity can be enhanced by several different mechanisms. These include structural alterations in the regulatory domains of the kinases (Coussens et al. 1986; Ullrich et al. 1984; Roussel et al. 1987), changes in the phosphorylation state of the kinases (Bertics and Gill 1985; Roussel et al. 1987; Yu and Czech 1986), and enhanced amounts of the tyrosine kinases. Most recently it has been directly shown that mere amplification of the HER-2 gene product causes transformation of cultured cells and tumorigenesis when these cells are injected into animals (Di Fiore et al. 1987; Hudziak et al. 1987). In addition, the HER-2 gene has been found to be amplified in 30% of pri-

Recent Results in Cancer Research, Vol. 113
© Springer-Verlag Berlin·Heidelberg 1989

mary human breast cancers. It is important that amplification of the gene is associated with disease relapse and overall patient survival (Slamon et al. 1987). Analyses of breast carcinoma cell lines indicate that as many as 60% of the tumor cells may have elevated expression of the HER-2 gene as a result of enhanced levels of transcription in addition to gene amplification (Kraus et al. 1987). Taken together, these studies suggest that overexpression of the HER-2 gene and possibly other members of the tyrosine kinase gene family may play a crucial role in the genesis and development of some types of human cancer. Moreover these findings provide new potential for diagnostic approaches.

There are several possible approaches toward cancer diagnosis based on the detection of amplified proto-oncogene or oncogene expression. One approach is to quantitate amplification of the gene, its transcripts, or protein product in the tumor tissue. While this approach is the most direct, it requires removal of tumor tissue from the patient in sufficient quantities for extraction and detection of specific DNA sequences, RNA transcripts or protein products that have not been degraded.

In this report we present an alternative approach toward possible cancer diagnosis on the basis of the detection of amplified tyrosine kinase activity in serum or plasma. Although tyrosine kinases are generally confined to the cell and are not known to be secreted, there are examples of the release of cellular proteins as well as tumor antigens into serum (Bellet et al. 1984; Gutman 1959). Additional evidence that cellular oncogene products are released from tumor cells comes from the known presence of circulating antibodies specific for several oncogene-coded proteins in the serum of tumor-bearing animals (Bishop 1985). In fact, the initial identification of retroviral oncogene products was obtained through the use of specific antibodies, produced in tumor-bearing rabbits, which were used to immunoprecipitate cellular oncogene products from transformed cells (Bishop 1985). Although these proteins are localized inside the cell, sufficient amounts were released from the tumor cells to elicit antibody production. We have focussed our efforts toward the detection of tyrosine kinases in serum as a possible diagnostic tool for several reasons. Firstly, most tyrosine kinases discovered to date are the products of proto-oncogenes and have been found to function in normal and malignant cell growth (Hunter and Cooper 1985). Since enhanced tyrosine kinase activity is associated with an uncontrolled growth of cells, tyrosine kinase levels may directly reflect the growth rate of the cells in the tumor. Secondly, assays for tyrosine kinase activity using phosphorylation of a substrate with $(\gamma\text{-}^{32}P)ATP$ are extremely sensitive. Thirdly, serum samples are easily obtained and can be repeatedly sampled to monitor changes in the expression of the proto-oncogene product that may reflect the growth rate of the tumor cells.

Experimental Procedures

Materials

Tumor-bearing rabbit sera were obtained from Dr. Herman Opperman. Sera from patients with malignant disorders were from Charity Hospital, New Orleans, LA, and from Dr. Bruce Dana, Department of Oncology, The Oregon Health Sciences

University, Portland, OR. Sera from apparently healthy individuals were from volunteers. All other materials were obtained from previously described sources (Lin et al. 1985, 1987).

Serum Tyrosine Protein Kinase Assay

The kinase reaction mixture contained 20 mM Hepes, 10 mM MnC12, 5 mM dithiothreitol, 0.5% Nonidet P-40, 25 μM sodium orthovanadate, 10 μM ATP, and 5 μCi [(γ-^{32}P]ATP. A quantity of 2.5 μl anti-src IgG that was preheated at 56 °C for 30 min was used as the substrate (Clinton et al. 1982). The reaction was incubated at 34 °C for 5 min and was stopped by the addition of an equal volume of twofold concentrated RIPA buffer (Lin et al. 1985, 1987). Then, 100 μl of a 50% suspension of protein A sepharose was incubated with the reaction mixture to bind the IgG substrate. The protein A sepharose complexed to the IgG was washed three times with RIPA buffer, suspended and boiled for 2 min in Laemmli gel electrophoresis sample buffer, and electrophoresed in a 10% polyacrylamide SDS-containing gel.

For serum kinase assays using angiotensin as the substrate, 200 μg angiotensin II in place of the anti-src IgG was added to the reaction mixture. The reaction was terminated by boiling for 3 min. Quantitation of phosphorylated angiotensin was by high-voltage paper electrophoresis exactly as described (Lin et al. 1985, 1987).

Results

Detection of proto-oncogene products with tyrosine kinase activity in serum samples requires that the protein is not rapidly cleared from the serum, that the kinase activity is preserved, and that the amount released from the tumor is sufficient to be detected in a reasonable quantity of serum. To explore the feasibility of serum assays we began our studies with sera from tumor-bearing rabbits that had been infected with Rous sarcoma virus and that contained antibodies to the oncogene encoded tyrosine kinase, pp60v-src. Sera from three separate tumor-bearing rabbits, infected with Rous sarcoma virus, were tested for tyrosine kinase activity and compared with normal, control rabbit serum. Of each sample 5 μl was incubated in a kinase reaction containing (γ-^{32}P)ATP and exogenous IgG was used for the tyrosine kinase substrate. This IgG, which is specific for pp60src, is phosphorylated by tyrosine kinases, but not serine or threonine kinases (Clinton et al. 1982). Figure 1 is an autoradiogram of the gel containing the phosphorylated products from the serum kinase reactions in which the position of migration of the IgG substrate is designated. The level of phosphorylation was from six- to twelvefold higher in three separate serum samples from tumor-bearing rabbits (Fig. 1, lanes B–D) compared with serum from a normal apparently healthy rabbit (Fig. 1, lane A). Although the anti-src IgG has been found to be a tyrosine kinase substrate, it was important to determine that the IgG was phosphorylated on tyrosine residues by serum enzymes. The phosphorylated IgG from the gel shown in Fig. 1 (lanes A, B, and C) was eluted from the gel, partially acid hydrolyzed, and the phosphoamino acids were resolved by paper electrophoresis. Only tyrosine was found to be phosphorylated (Fig. 2). The amount of phosphotyrosine was proportional to the level of phosphorylation of IgG (Fig. 1) verifying that there was more tyrosine phosphorylation activity in the tumor-bearing rabbit sera compared with the normal rabbit serum. Elevations in the tyrosine kinase activity in the tumor-bearing rabbit sera were also observed when other substrates were used in the kinase reaction. These included the peptide angiotensin and a glutamic acid-tyrosine polymer (data not shown).

To test whether the elevated tyrosine kinase was from the viral src gene, the anti-src IgG, which recognizes viral but not cellular pp60src (Clinton et al. 1982), was caused to react with the different sera, and the immune complex was washed several times to remove contaminating proteins prior to assaying for kinase activity. IgG was phosphorylated in the washed immune complex providing evidence that the elevated kinase activity in the tumor-bearing rabbit sera was from the Rous sarcoma virus oncogene. These results provided the first indication that a cellular oncogene protein is released from tumors and retains its kinase activity in serum. Moreover, the assay was sufficiently sensitive to detect kinase activity in 5 µl or less of tumor-bearing rabbit sera.

Because we were able to detect the viral-src oncogene product with tyrosine kinase activity in small amounts of tumor-bearing rabbit sera, we were encouraged to begin investigations of tyrosine kinase levels in sera from patients with malignant disorders. When these studies were initiated, it was not known which type of human tumor was likely to contain elevated levels of a tyrosine kinase. Therefore, serum samples were collected from patients with a variety of malignant disorders

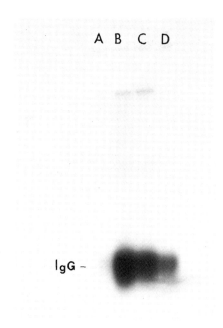

Fig. 1. Tyrosine kinase activity in tumor-bearing rabbit sera. Quantities of 5 µl sera from tumor-bearing rabbits that had been infected with Rous sarcoma virus *(lanes B, C,* and *D)* and serum from an uninfected rabbit *(lane A)* were incubated in a kinase reaction. The ^{32}P-labelled IgG was localized by protein staining of the gels and autoradiography

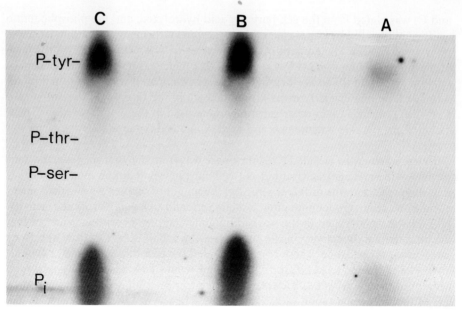

Fig. 2. Amino acids phosphorylated in anti-src IgG by rabbit sera. The ³²P-labelled IgG phosphorylated in the serum kinase reaction shown in Fig. 1 was cut from the gel and eluted by electrophoresis. The eluted protein was partially acid-hydrolyzed and analyzed by high-voltage paper electrophoresis at pH 3.5 as previously described (Clinton et al. 1982). The phosphoamino acid markers were detected by ninhydrin staining and the ³²P-labelled material was localized by autoradiography. *A, B,* and *C* correspond to the lanes in Fig. 1

who had not recently undergone surgery, as well as from cancer-free individuals. A kinase assay was conducted with 5 µl human serum exactly as described in Fig. 1 using anti-src IgG as the substrate. Autoradiography of the gel containing the product of the reaction, phosphorylated IgG, is shown in Fig. 3 where lanes A–F contain the product phosphorylated by patient's sera and lanes G–L contain the product phosphorylated by control sera. This initial screening indicated that a patient with malignant melanoma (Fig. 3 A) revealed serum tyrosine kinase activity that was from four to ten times higher than that of the other individuals who were tested.

To indicate the proportion of the patients with malignant melanoma who may have elevated tyrosine kinase activity, several serum samples were collected. Each of the twelve samples from patients with malignant melanoma was matched with a control sample from an individual of the same age and sex, and the two were assayed. In each case, the tyrosine kinase activities were determined in 5 µl serum using the peptide angiotensin as the substrate (Lin et al. 1985). Quantitations of the tyrosine-specific protein kinase activity revealed that in ten of the twelve matched pairs, the patients with malignant melanoma had higher levels of activity (Table 1).

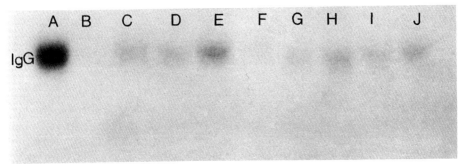

Fig. 3. Tyrosine kinase activity in human sera. Human sera (5 µl) was incubated in a kinase reaction, and the product was analyzed by SDS-gel electrophoresis exactly as in Fig. 1. The ^{32}P-labelled IgG was detected by autoradiography of the gel. *Lanes A-F* designate the samples from individuals with malignant disorders. *Lanes G-J* designate the samples from apparently healthy individuals

Table 1. Tyrosine kinase activity (µmol/min/ml serum)

Group	Control	Melanoma	Fold increase
1	139	354	2.6
2	189	468	2.5
3	280	1680	6.0
4	239	306	1.3
5	178	276	1.6
6	224	119	0.5
7	104	85	0.8
8	114	241	2.1
9	118	128	1.1
10	148	198	1.3
11	108	206	1.9
12	160	214	1.3

Serum samples were obtained from patients with malignant melanoma. These patients have metastatic disease and had not undergone recent surgery. The patients' samples were each matched with serum samples from apparently healthy individuals of the same sex and within two years of the same age. The paired samples were assayed for 2.5 min in a kinase reaction containing angiotensin as the substrate. The ^{32}P-labelled phosphorylated angiotensin was quantitated (Lin et al. 1985, 1987) and the tyrosine kinase activity was calculated as the µmoles of phosphate transferred to angiotensin per minute per milliliter of serum.

Discussion

In the present study, pp60src with tyrosine kinase activity was detected in 5 µl or less of sera from three separate tumor-bearing rabbits that had been infected with Rous sarcoma virus. The antibodies used to assay the serum samples react with viral but not cellular pp60src (Clinton et al. 1982), indicating that the elevated kinase in the serum was most likely a product of the viral oncogene. Although pp60src is a cytoplasmic protein, sufficient quantities were apparently released from tumor cells to allow detection of the enzyme in very small amounts of sera. These results with sera from tumor-bearing rabbits suggested the possibility of monitoring the expression of protooncogene products, particularly those with tyrosine kinase activity, in serum samples from patients with malignant disorders. A serum assay for protooncogene products has potential value as a diagnostic tool.

Preliminary screening of ten human samples showed that a patient with malignant melanoma had the highest serum tyrosine kinase activity. Moreover, this elevation was observed in twelve of fourteen samples from patients with malignant melanoma who were randomly paired with age- and sex-matched control samples from apparently healthy individuals. Although the elevations in serum tyrosine kinase levels appear to be significant, the magnitude of the elevation over that of apparently normal individuals may not be sufficient for clinical diagnosis of malignant melanoma. Assays of a specific tyrosine kinase that may be elevated exclusively in the melanoma cells may provide a more sensitive screening procedure.

One difficulty with the development of assays of tumor-derived tyrosine kinases is that there is a surprisingly high level of background tyrosine kinase activity in sera from normal individuals. The tyrosine kinase activity is found in a soluble form in both serum and plasma and the amount of activity is variable from individual to individual (Lin et al. 1985). One factor that appears to affect serum tyrosine kinase activity is the age of the individual. In a study conducted on over 200 samples, the cord blood from newborns appeared to have significantly higher levels of tyrosine kinase activity than sera from individuals of up to 20 years of age (Lin et al. 1987). With increasing age, the individual variability obscured attempts to define age-related effects. Thus efforts to assign a control or normal serum tyrosine kinase level to be used as a standard have been thwarted by the presence of high and variable levels of serum tyrosine kinase activity, particularly in individuals who are older than 30 years.

Future prospects for development of a serum assay of prognostic value will most likely involve measurements of specific tyrosine kinases that are released from tumor cells. Recent findings that the HER-2 protein is amplified in a large proportion of breast cancer cells (Kraus et al. 1987; Slamon et al. 1987) suggested the possibility of assaying this specific tyrosine kinase in serum. In a preliminary screening of eight samples from patients with stage 3 or stage 4 breast adenocarcinoma, we have been unable to detect significantly elevated HER-2 protein either by immunoblotting or by immunoprecipitation of self-phosphorylated protein. It is possible that the transmembrane proto-oncogene products such as the HER-2 protein remain in membrane complexes and are rapidly cleared from the serum, while the cytoplasmic proto-oncogene products such as pp60src are released in a soluble form where the kinase activity can be detected in the serum.

References

Bellet DH, Wands JR, Isselbacher KJ, Bohuon C (1984) Serum α-fetoprotein levels in human disease: perspective from a highly specific monoclonal radioimmunoassay. Proc Natl Acad Sci USA 81: 3869–3873

Bertics PJ, Gill SN (1985) Self-phosphorylation enhances the protein-tyrosine kinase activity of the epidermal growth factor receptor. J Biol Chem 260: 14642–14647

Bishop JM (1983) Cellular oncogenes and retroviruses. Ann Rev Biochem 52: 301–354

Brodeur GM, Seeger RC, Schwab M, Varmus HE, Bishop JM (1984) Amplification of N-*myc* in untreated human neuroblastomas correlates with advanced disease stage. Science 224: 1121–1124

Clinton GM, Guerina NG, Guo H-Y, Huang AS (1982) Host-dependent phosphorylation and kinase activity associated with vesicular stomatitis virus. J Biol Chem 257: 3313–3319

Coussens L, van Beveren C, Smith D, Chen E, Mitchell RL, Isake CM, Verma IM, Ullrich A (1986) Structural alteration of viral homologue of receptor protooncogene *fms* at carboxyl terminus. Nature 320: 277–280

Di Fiore PP, Pierce JH, Kraus MH, Segatto O, King CR, Aaronson SA (1987) Erb-B-2 is a potent oncogene when overexpressed in NIH/3T3 cells. Science 237: 778–781

Downward J, Yarden Y, Mayes E, Scarce G, Totty N, Stockwell P, Ullrich A, Schlessinger J, Waterfield MD (1984) Close similarity of epidermal growth factor receptor and V-erb-B oncogene protein sequences. Nature 307: 521–527

Gutman AB (1959) Serum alkaline phosphatase activity in diseases of the skeletal and hepatobiliary systems. Am J Med 27: 875–901

Hudziak RM, Schlessinger J, Ullrich A (1987) Increased expression of the putative growth factor receptor p185^{HER2} causes transformation and tumorogenesis of NIH/3T3 cells. Proc Natl Acad Sci USA 84: 7159–7163

Hunter T, Cooper JA (1985) Protein-tyrosine kinases. Ann Rev Biochem 54: 897–930

Kraus MH, Popescu NC, Amsbaugh SC, King CR (1987) Overexpression of the EGF receptor related protooncogene erb B-2 in human mammary tumor cell lines by different molecular mechanisms. EMBO J 6: 605–610

Lin M-F, Lee P, Clinton GM (1985) Characterization of tyrosyl kinase activity in human serum. J Biol Chem 260: 1582–1587

Lin M-F, Bailey-Wilson JE, Elston RC, Clinton GM (1987) Developmental expression of tyrosyl kinase activity in human serum. Hum Biol 59: 549–556

Padhy LC, Shih C, Cowing D, Finkelstein R, Weinberg RA (1982) Identification of a phosphoprotein specifically induced by the transforming DNA of rat neuroblastomas. Cell 28: 865–871

Rosen OM, Herrera R, Olowe Y, Petruzelli LM, Cobb MH (1983) Phosphorylation activates the insulin receptor tyrosine protein kinase. Proc Natl Acad Sci USA 80: 3237–3240

Roussel MF, Dull TJ, Rettenmier CW, Ralph P, Ullrich A, Sherr CJ (1987) Transforming potential of the C-*fms* protooncogene (CSF-1 receptor). Nature 325: 549–552

Schecter AL, Stern DF, Vaidyanathan L, Decker SJ, Drebin JA, Greene MI, Weinberg RA (1984) The *neu* oncogene an erb-B-related gene encoding a 185,000-Mr tumor antigen. Nature 312: 513–516

Sherr CJ, Rettenmier CW, Sacca R, Roussel MF, Cook AT, Stanley ER (1985) The C-*fms* proto-oncogene product is related to the receptor for the mononuclear phagocyte factor, CSF-1. Cell 41: 665–676

Slamon DJ, Clark GM, Wong SG, Levin WJ, Ullrich A, McGuire WL (1987) Human breast cancer: correlation of relapse and survival with amplification of the HER-2/neu oncogene. Science 235: 177–181

Ullrich A, Coussens L, Hayblick JS, Dull TJ, Gray A, Tam AW, Lee J, Yarden Y, Libermann TA, Schlessinger J, Downward J, Mayes ELV, Whittle N, Waterfield MD, Seeburg PH (1984) Human epidermal growth factor receptor cDNA sequence and aberrant expression of the amplified gene in A431 epidermoid carcinoma cells. J Biol Chem 261: 4715–4722

Xu YH, Richert N, Ito S, Merlino GT, Pastan I (1984) Characterization of epidermal growth factor receptor gene expression in malignant and normal human cell lines. Proc Natl Acad Sci USA 81: 7308–7312

Yarden Y, Escobedo JA, Kuang W-J, Yang-Feng TL, Daniel TO, Tremble PM, Chen EY, Ando ME, Harkins RN, Francke U, Fried VA, Ullrich A, Williams LT (1986) Structure of the receptor for platelet-derived growth factor helps define a family of closely related growth factor receptors. Nature 323: 226–232

Yu KT, Czech MP (1985) Tyrosine phosphorylation of insulin receptor beta subunit activates the receptor tyrosine kinase in intact H-35 hepatoma cells. J Biol Chem 261: 4715–4722

Ribosomal Protein S6 Kinase and PKC in Human Mammary Tumor Cells*

D. Fabbro[1], I. Novak-Hofer[1], W. Küng[1], T. Meyer[2], A. Matter[2], and U. Eppenberger[1]

[1] Laboratorien, Kantonsspital Basel, Universitäts-Frauenklinik, 4031 Basel, Switzerland
[2] CiBA-GEIGY, 4002 Basel, Switzerland

Introduction

It is well established that 17-β estradiol (E_2) influences the growth of human breast cancer (Patterson et al. 1982; Edwards et al. 1979; Maass and Jonat 1983; Howat et al. 1985), but it is unclear wheter E_2 acts directly or indirectly on the proliferation of target cells (Soto and Sonnenschein 1987; Dickson and Lippman 1987; King 1985). At present, there is increasing evidence that polypeptide growth factors (GF) also regulate the growth of human breast cancer (Dickson and Lippman 1987; King 1985; Dickson et al. 1986; Dickson et al. 1986). Therefore, E_2 may in part promote the growth through the regulation of autostimulatory and autoinhibitory GFs (Soto and Sonnenschein 1987; Dickson and Lippman 1987; Knabbe et al. 1987). Consequently, the hormone dependency of breast tumor cells may be limited not only to functional estrogen receptors (ER) but also to functional growth factor receptors (GF-R). Such GF-Rs are likely to represent important growth-regulatory elements in the estrogen-induced autocrine or paracrine growth mechanisms of human breast cancer (Fitzpatrick et al. 1984; Macias et al. 1986; Sainsbury et al. 1985; Wyss et al. 1987; Sainsbury et al. 1987; Furlanetto and DiCarlo 1984).

Transduction of extracellular GF signals into a mitogenic program involves a variety of protein kinases (Hunter 1987). For example, the cytoplasmic tyrosine protein kinase (TyrPK) of the receptors for epidermal growth factor (EGF), platelet-derived growth factor (PDGF), insulin and somatomedin C (SMC) are rapidly stimulated following the binding of GFs to their respective GF-Rs (Cohen et al. 1980; Ek et al. 1982; Jacobs et al. 1983; Kasuga et al. 1982). The activation of GF-Rs also results in the rapid stimulation of an S6-kinase (S6-PK), which specifically phosphorylates the S6 protein located on the small 40s ribosomal subunit (Thomas et al. 1979; Novak-Hofer and Thomas 1984; Novak-Hofer and Thomas 1985; Tabarini et al. 1985; Blenis and Erikson 1985). The activation of S6-PK has been coupled to the initiation of DNA synthesis because a variety of growth-promoting agents such as serum, GFs, and tumor promoters stimulate S6 phosphorylation (Novak-Hofer and Thomas 1984; Novak-Hofer and Thomas 1985; Tabarini et al.

* This study was supported in part by the Swiss National Foundation Number 3.344-0.86 and the Roche Research Foundation (I. N.).

1985; Blenis and Erikson 1985). The binding of GFs to their GF-Rs also results in the formation of diacylglycerol and Ca^{2+}, which stimulate in concert the multifunctional protein kinase C (PKC), the major receptor for tumor-promoting phorbol esters (Berridge and Irvine 1984; Nishizuka 1984; Nishizuka 1986).

How the activation of these protein kinases eventually leads to the onset of a mitogenic program remains unclear, but it is conceivable that they play an important regulatory role in signal transduction (Hunter 1987). The understanding of their mechanisms of action may help to discriminate better between hormone-dependent and hormone-independent breast tumor growth and may in future open new avenues for pharmaceutical intervention.

Results

Effects of E_2 and GFs on S6-PK and the Growth of Human Mammary Tumor Cells

The natural history of human breast tumors often involves the transition from an E_2-responsive to a more aggressive E_2-unresponsive phenotype (Patterson et al. 1982; Edwards et al. 1979; Maass and Jonat 1983; Howat et al. 1985). Both E_2-dependent and E_2-independent breast tumors can be studied in tissue culture using a set of established human breast cancer cells (Cailleau et al. 1974; Horwitz et al. 1978; Engel and Young 1978). They can be subdivided into cells containing the ER (ER positive), which display an obligate E_2 requirement for growth as well as tumor formation, such as ZR-75, and into cells lacking the ER (ER negative), which are independent of E_2 for growth in vivo and in vitro, such as MDA-MB-231 (Engel and Young 1978). Under strictly controlled conditions, free of serum and phenol red (Küng et al. 1986; Berthois et al. 1986), the growth of the ZR-75

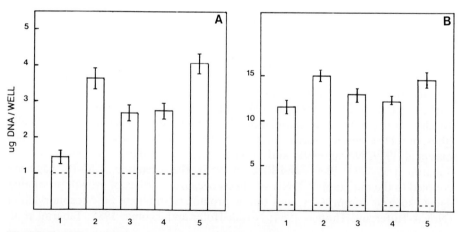

Fig. 1A, B. Effect of GFs and E_2 on the growth of ZR-75 cells (**A**) and MDA-MB-231 cells (**B**). Cells were grown under serum-free conditions (Küng et al. 1986), and DNA was determined 9 days after addition of various agents (Roos et al. 1986). *Dotted lines* indicate seeding densities. *1,* control; *2,* 500 n*M* insulin; *3,* 3 n*M* E_2; *4,* 1 n*M* EGF; *5,* 10 n*M* SMC

cells is not only stimulated by E_2 but also by α-TGF, EGF and SMC (Fig. 1 A), whereas the MDA-MB-231 cells are stimulated neither by E_2 nor by any of the GFs tested (Fig. 1 B). Nevertheless, all human mammary tumor cells contain receptors for SMC, insulin (Furlanetto and DiCarlo 1984; Osborn et al. 1978), and EGF (Roos et al. 1986). The stimulation of serum-deprived ZR-75 and MDA-MB-231 cells with fetal calf serum (FCS) or EGF revealed that EGF, as well as other GFs, were not able to activate S6-PK of MDA-MB-231 cells (Fig. 2). This lack of EGF-dependent activation is not due to a nonfunctional S6-PK in MDA-MB-231 cells, since mitogenic factors in the FCS were able to activate S6-PK in these cells (Fig. 2). In contrast, activation of the S6-PK by EGF or FCS in the ZR-75 cell line occurred to a similar extent (Fig. 2). Maximal activation was achieved 30 min after the addition of the EGF homolog, α-TGF, or EGF to ZR-75 cells and decreased thereafter correlating with the down-regulation of the EGF-R (Novak-Hofer et al.

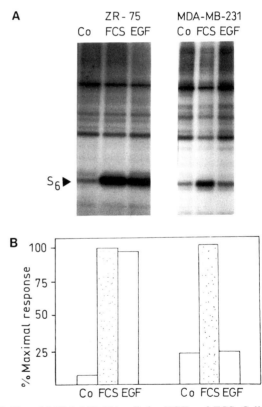

Fig. 2 A, B. Activation of S6-PK of ZR-75 and MDA-MB-231 cells by EGF and FCS. Cell extracts of serum-starved cells stimulated for 30 min with FCS (15% final) and 10 n M EGF were incubated with 40s ribosomal subunits and γ-[^{32}P]ATP followed by separation of the phosphoproteins on 15%-SDS polyacrylamide gels and autoradiography (Novak-Hofer and Thomas 1984). **A** Autoradiograms. The *arrow* marks the S6 protein. **B** Quantitation of S6-phosphorylation. *Co,* control; *EGF,* stimulated with 10 n M EGF (30 min); *FCS,* stimulated with 15% FCS (30 min)

1987). Stimulation of S6-PK by EGF or α-TGF cells was dose-dependent (Fig. 3) closely matching the amounts of GF required for half-maximal stimulation of growth of ZR-75 cells (Novak-Hofer et al. 1987). No increase of S6-PK activity was, however, observed with E_2 in ZR-75 cells at any dose and time of incubation tested (Fig. 3).

Role of PKC in the Growth Regulation of Human Mammary Tumor Cells

There is evidence for a possible involvement of PKC in the growth regulation of human breast cancer cells. Pronounced effects on growth, morphology, and PKC are observed upon the addition of tumor promoters such as 12-O-tetradecanoyl-phorbol-13-acetate (TPA) to human breast tumor cells (Roos et al. 1986; Regazzi et al. 1986). Growth resumption upon removal of TPA coincided with the reappearance of the TPA–down-regulated PKC activity in the MCF-7 cell line (Fabbro et al. 1986a). Moreover, an inverse relationship between the levels of PKC and ER was found in tissue culture (Fabbro et al. 1986b; Borner et al. 1987) or mammary tumor biopsies (Wyss et al. 1987) (Fig. 4). The S6-PK of ZR-75 cells is stimulated by TPA, EGF, SMC, or high levels of insulin (Fig. 5A). No TPA-dependent activation of S6-PK occurred, however, when PKC activity was previously down-regulated by prolonged TPA-pretreatement (Fig. 5B), whereas EGF, insulin, or SMC

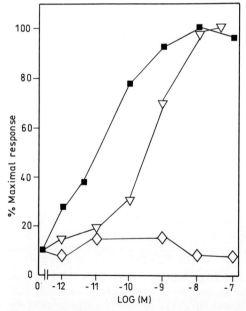

Fig. 3. Effects of EGF, α-TGF, and E_2 on S6-PK of ZR-75 cells. Serum-deprived ZR-75 cells were exposed to increasing concentrations of E_2 for 1 h or to increasing doses of α-TGF or EGF for 30 min followed by determination and quantitation of S6-PK activity as described in legend to Fig. 2. $\diamond$, E_2; ■, EGF; $\triangledown$, α-TGF

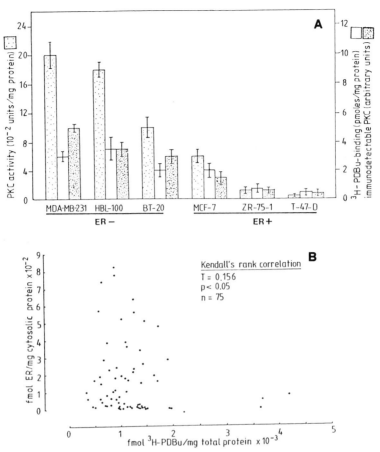

Fig. 4A, B. Quantitative relationship between PKC and ER in human mammary tumor biopsies **A** or tissue culture **B**. Quantitation of PKC by phorbol ester binding, protein kinase activity, and PKC immunodetection in tissue culture, as well as determination of PKC and ER in human mammary tumor biopsies were performed as described. (Borner et al. 1987; Wyss et al. 1987)

led to a similar increase in S6-PK activity irrespective of the prolonged pretreatment of ZR-75 cells by TPA (Fig. 5 B). These data suggest that stimulation of S6-PK by GFs also occurs in the absence of PKC activity and indicates the presence of additional GF-signalling pathway(s) bypassing PKC. Therefore, the presence of PKC-dependent and PKC-independent pathways should be considered if inhibition of the PKs that are involved in GF-mediated signal transduction is attempted.

Several PKC inhibitors (Hannun et al. 1986; Tamaoki et al. 1986; Kase et al. 1986) are commercially available, but no inhibitor of S6-PK has yet been described. Except for staurosporine (Tamaoki et al. 1986), all PKC inhibitors display inhibitory activity only within a micromolar range with marginal effects on cell growth. Staurosporine not only inhibited partially purified PKC but also purified

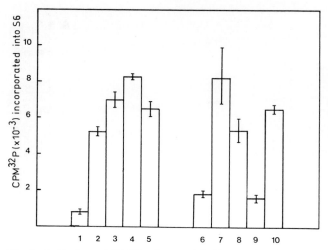

Fig. 5. Activation of S6-PK of control *(left)* and of TPA-treated ZR-75 *(right)* cells. Serum-starved ZR-75 cells *(1–5)* or ZR-75 cells pretreated with 300 nM TPA for 48 h *(6–10)* were exposed for 30 min to vehicle *(1, 6)*, 10 nM EGF *(2, 7)*, 1000 nM insulin *(3, 8)*, 300 nM TPA *(4, 9)*, and 10 nM SMC *(5, 10)*, followed by determination and quantitation of S6-PK activity. Results are expressed as means ± SD ($n = 2$)

S6-PK in a dose-dependent manner with IC_{50} of 3 nM and 20 nM respectively (Fig. 6 A). In addition, half-maximal inhibition for the EGF- or TPA-dependent activation of S6-PK occurred at staurosporine concentrations of 100 nM and 10 nM respectively in intact ZR-75 cells (Fig. 6 B). Thus, the difference in the IC_{50} of staurosporine required to inhibit PKC and S6-PK in the test tube corresponded well to the IC_{50} of staurosporine for the inhibition of the TPA- and EGF-dependent activation of S6-PK in intact cells (Figs. 6 A and 6 B). Interestingly, exposure of either ER-positive or ER-negative human mammary tumor cells to increasing doses of staurosporine for 4 days also resulted in a growth inhibition (Fig. 6 C). Half-maximal inhibition of growth occurred at doses of staurosporine that are required to half-maximally inhibit PKC and S6-PK (Fig. 6).

Discussion

In contrast to the GF-activated DNA synthesis, the E_2-stimulated proliferation is not well characterized (Soto and Sonnenschein 1987; Dickson and Lippman 1987). Since in mammary tumor cells, E_2 increases the production of GFs such as the EGF homolog α-TGF and SMC (Dickson and Lippman 1987; Dickson et al. 1986a; Dickson et al. 1986b), an autocrine growth regulation of breast cancer cells has been proposed (Dickson and Lippman 1987). Consequently, E_2 should also trigger molecular responses characteristic for GFs. In contrast to EGF and SMC, however, E_2 did not increase S6-PK activity in ZR-75 cells, a typical response to many GFs (Novak-Hofer and Thomas 1984; Novak-Hofer and Thomas 1985; Tabarini et al. 1985; Blenis and Erikson 1985), although S6-PK activation by EGF or

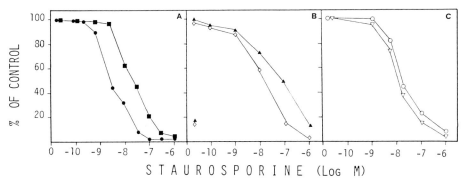

Fig. 6A–C. Effect of staurosporine on the S6-PK activation. **A** Highly purified pig brain PKC (Borner et al. 1987) or highly purified S6-PK from 3T3 fibroblasts (Jenö et al. 1988) were exposed to increasing concentrations of staurosporine. Results are expressed as % of protein kinase inhibition. ●, PKC; ■, S6-PK. **B** Serum-deprived ZR-75 cells were incubated for 30 min with either 10 nM EGF (▲) or 100 nM TPA (◇) in the presence of increasing concentrations of staurosporine, followed by quantitation of S6-PK activity. Results are expressed as % of maximal activity. *Symbols on the left corner of panel B* show basal activity in the absence of EGF or TPA. **C** The ER-positive MCF-7 (▽) and the ER-negative MDA-MB-231 (○) cells were exposed for 4 days to increasing concentrations of staurosporine followed by determination of DNA

α-TGF in ZR-75 cells exhibited a dose-response curve similar to that found for growth stimulated by EGF or α-TGF (Novak-Hofer et al. 1987). Since E_2 bypasses the activation of S6-PK and S6 phosphorylation (Novak-Hofer et al. 1987), our results do not support the hypothesis of a stimulation of ZR-75 cell growth via an E_2-dependent production of α-TGF.

However, hormone-independent mammary tumor cells also produce α-TGF and SMC (Dickson and Lippman 1987; Dickson et al. 1986a; Dickson et al. 1986b). Surprisingly, MDA-MB-231 cells, which are not growth stimulated by EGF and SMC, did not exhibit a GF-dependent S6-PK activation, although these cells contain a functional S6-PK. It appears, therefore, that only the ER-positive cells have conserved a GF-dependent growth regulation and the inability of GFs to stimulate proliferation of ER-negative cells is also reflected in the lack of S6-PK activation. Specifically, the EGF-dependent activation of S6-PK in ER-positive cells apparently relies on functional high-affinity EGF-Rs (Roos et al. 1986; Fabbro et al. 1986b). Thus, the GF production of hormone-independent (ER-negative) mammary tumor cells may play a role in paracrine rather than autocrine growth stimulation.

Down-regulation of PKC activity by long-term treatment with TPA (Regazzi et al. 1986; Fabbro et al. 1986a) blocked the activation of S6-PK by TPA in ZR-75 cells, although EGF, SMC, and insulin also stimulated S6-PK in the absence of PKC. It is now well established that S6-PK is different than PKC (Tabarini et al. 1985; Blenis and Erikson 1985; Novak-Hofer and Thomas 1985). However, in the case of TPA, a functional PKC is required to stimulate S6-PK (Tabarini et al. 1985; Blenis and Erikson 1985). The mechanisms by which GFs and TPA stimulate S6-PK are unknown, but phosphorylation of S6-PK appears to be required for its activation (Novak-Hofer and Thomas 1985; Ballou et al. 1988). To better discriminate between the TPA- and GF-dependent activation of S6-PK the PKC inhibitor staurosporine (Tamaoki et al. 1986) was used. This compound effectively inhibited the activation of S6-PK by EGF and TPA in intact ZR-75 cells, although with a different IC_{50} coinciding with the IC_{50} for the inhibition in the test tube of purified PKC and S6-PK. Staurosporine has been shown to inhibit PKC by affecting its protein kinase activity (Tamaoki et al. 1986). Interestingly, staurosporine also inhibited the proliferation of human breast cancer cells irrespective of the presence of ER.

In conclusion, our results support the hypothesis that different pathways are involved in the transduction of the GF signal that ultimately leads to the activation of the S6-PK. Therefore, inhibition of the protein kinases that play a role in signal transduction, such as PKC, S6-PK, and the TyrPKs of GF-Rs, may also result in the inhibition of cellular growth and may lead, in future, to the development of compounds that allow a better management of human breast cancer.

Acknowledgements. We are greatly indebted to P.Jenö and G.Thomas for the purified S6 kinase. Staurosporine was provided by Ciba-Geigy, Basel. The excellent technical assistance of I.Lützelschwab and E.Silber is appreciated.

References

Ballou LM, Jenö P, Thomas G (1988) Protein phosphatase 2A inactivates the mitogen-stimulated S6 kinase from Swiss mouse 3T3 cells. J Biol Chem 263: 1188–1194

Berridge MJ, Irvine RF (1984) Inositol trisphosphate, a novel second messenger in cellular signal transduction. Nature 312: 315–321

Berthois Y, Katzenellenbogen JA, Katzenellenbogen BS (1986) Phenol red in tissue culture media is a weak estrogen implications concerning the study of estrogen-responsive cells in culture. Proc Natl Acad Sci USA 83: 2496–2500

Blenis J, Erikson R (1985) Regulation of a ribosomal protein S6 kinase by the rous sarcoma virus transforming protein, serum and phorbol ester. Proc Natl Acad Sci USA 82: 7621–7625

Borner C, Wyss R, Regazzi R, Eppenberger U, Fabbro D (1987) Immunological quantitation of phospholipid/Ca^{2+}-dependent protein kinase of human mammary carcinoma cells: Inverse relationship to estrogen receptors. Int J Cancer 40: 344–348

Cailleau R, Young R, Olive M, Reeves WJ (1974) Breast tumor cell lines from pleural effusions. J Natl Cancer Inst 53: 661–667

Cohen S, Carpenter G, King L (1980) Epidermal growth factor receptor protein kinase interactions. J Biol Chem 255: 4834–4842

Dickson RB, Bates SE, McManaway ME, Lippman ME (1986) Characterization of estrogen responsive transforming activity in human breast cancer cell lines. Cancer Res 46: 1707–1713

Dickson RB, McManaway ME, Lippman ME (1986) Estrogen-induced factors of breast cancer cells partially replace estrogen to promote tumor growth. Science 232: 1540–1543

Dickson RB, Lippman ME (1987) Estrogenic regulation of growth and polypeptide growth factor secretion in human breast cancer carcinoma. Endocrine Rev 8: 29–43

Edwards DP, Chamness GC, McGuire WL (1979) Estrogen and progesterone receptor proteins in breast cancer. Biochem Biophys Acta 560: 457–468

Engel WL, Young NA (1978) Human breast carcinoma cells in continuous culture: A review, Cancer Res 38: 4327–4339

Ek B, Westermark B, Wasteson A, Heldin C (1982) Stimulation of tyrosine-specific phosphorylation by platelet-derived growth factor. Nature 295: 419–420

Fabbro D, Regazzi R, Costa SD, Borner C, Eppenberger U (1986a) Protein kinase C desensitization by phorbolesters and its impact on growth of human breast cancer cells. Biochem Biophys Res Commun 135: 65–73

Fabbro D, Küng W, Roos W, Regazzi R, Eppenberger U (1986b) Epidermal growth factor binding and protein kinase C activities in human Breast cancer cell lines: possible quantitative relationship. Cancer Res 46: 2720–2725

Fitzpatrick SL, Brightwell J, Wittliff JL, Barrows GH, Schultz GS (1984) Epidermal growth factor binding by breast tumor biopsies and relationship to estrogen receptor and progestin receptor levels. Cancer Res 44: 3448–3452

Furlanetto RW, DiCarlo JN (1984) Somatomedin C receptors and growth effects in human breast cells maintained in long-term tissue culture. Cancer Res 44: 2122–2128

Hannun YA, Loomis CR, Merrill AH Jr, Bell RM (1986) Sphingosine inhibition of protein kinase C activity and phorbol dibutyrate binding in vitro and in human platelets. J Biol Chem 261: 12604–12609

Horowitz KH, Zava DT, Arulasanam KT, Jensen EM, McGuire WL (1987) Steroid receptor analysis of nine human breast cancer cell lines. Cancer Res 38: 2434–2437

Howat JMT, Harris M, Swindell R, Barnes DM (1985) The effect of estrogen and progesterone receptors on recurrence and survival in patients with carcinoma of the breast. Br J Cancer 51: 263–270

Hunter T (1987) A thousand and one protein kinases. Cell 50: 823–829

Jacobs S, Kull FC Jr, Earp HS, Svoboda ME, Van Wyk JJ, Cuatrecasas P (1983) Somatomedin-C stimulates the phosphorylation of the beta-subunit of its own receptor. J Biol Chem 258: 9581–9584

Jenö P, Ballou LM, Novak-Hofer I, Thomas G (1988) Identification and characterization of a mitogen-activated S6 kinase. Proc Natl Acad Sci USA 85: 406–410

Kase H, Iwahashi K, Nakanishi S, Matsuda Y, Yamada K, Takahashi M, Murakata C, Sato A, Kaneko M (1986) K-252 compound a novel and potent inhibitor of protein kinase C and cyclic nucleotide-dependent protein kinases. Biochem Biophys Res Commun 142: 436–440

Kasuga M, Fujita-Yamaguchi Y, Blithe DL, Kahn CR (1982) Tyrosine specific protein kinase activity is associated with the purified insulin receptor. Proc Natl Acad Sci USA 80: 2137–2141

King RJB (1985) In: Cavalli F (ed) Endocrine Therapy of Breast Cancer: Experimental strategies for studying the development of breast cancer with special reference to steroid hormones, growth factors and oncogenes. Springer, Berlin Heidelberg New York Tokyo, pp 5–26

Knabbe C, Lippman ME, Wakefield LM, Flanders KC, Kasid A, Derynck R, Dickson RB (1987) Evidence that transforming growth factor-β is a hormonally regulated negative growth factor in human breast cancer cells. Cell 48: 417–428

Küng W, Silber E, Novak-Hofer I, Eppenberger U (1986) Effects of hormones and growth factors on the growth of six human breast cancer cell lines in defined media. In: Eppenberger U, Fabbro D, Schäfer P (eds) Contributions to oncology, vol. 23. Karger, Basel, pp 26–32

Maass H, Jonat W (1983) Steroid receptors as a guide for the therapy of primary and metastatic breast cancer. J Steroid Biochem 19: 833–837

Macias A, Azavedo E, Perez R, Rutqvist LE, Skoog L (1986) Receptors for epidermal growth factor in human mammary carcinomas and their metastases. Anticancer Res 6: 849–853

Nishizuka Y (1984) The role of protein kinase C in cell surface signal transduction and tumor promotion. Nature 308: 693–698

Nishizuka Y (1986) Studies and perspectives of protein kinase C. Science 233: 305–312

Novak-Hofer I, Thomas G (1984) An activated S6 kinase in extracts from serum and epidermal growth factor-stimulated Swiss 3T3 cells. J Biol Chem 259: 5995–6000

Novak-Hofer I, Thomas G (1985) Epidermal growth factor-mediated activation of an S6 kinase in Swiss mouse 3T3 cells. J Biol Chem 260: 10314–10319

Novak-Hofer I, Küng W, Fabbro D, Eppenberger U (1987) Estrogen stimulates growth of mammary tumor cells ZR-75 without activation of S6 kinase and S6 phosphorylation: difference from epidermal growth factor and α-transforming growth factor-induced proliferation. Eur J Biochem 164: 445–451

Osborn CK, Monaco ME, Lippman ME, Kahn CR (1978) Correlation among insulin binding, degradation and biological activity in human breast cancer cells in long term tissue culture. Cancer Res 38: 94–102

Patterson JS, Battersby LA, Edwards DG (1982) Review of the clinical pharmacology and international experience with tamoxifen in advanced breast cancer. In: Iacobelli S, (ed) The role of tamoxifen in breast cancer. Raven, New York, p 17

Regazzi R, Fabbro D, Costa SD, Borner C, Eppenberger U (1986) Effects of tumor promoters on growth and on cellular redistribution of phospholipid/Ca^{2+}-dependent protein kinase in human breast cancer cells. Int J Cancer 37: 731–737

Roos W, Fabbro D, Küng W, Costa SD, Eppenberger U (1986) Correlation between hormone dependency and the regulation of epidermal growth factor receptor by tumor promoters in human mammary carcinoma cells. Proc Natl Acad Sci USA 83: 991–995

Sainsbury JRC, Farndon JR, Sherbet GV, Harris AL (1985) Epidermal growth factor receptors and oestrogen receptors in human breast cancer. Lancet: 364–366

Sainsbury JRC, Farndon JR, Needham GK, Malcolm AJ, Harris AL (1987) Epidermal growth factor receptor status as predictor of early recurrence of and death from breast cancer. Lancet: 1398–1402

Soto AM, Sonnenschein C (1987) Cell proliferation of estrogen-sensitive cells: The case for negative control. Endocr Rev 8: 44–53

Tabarini D, Heinrich J, Rosen O (1985) Activation of S6 kinase activity in 3T3-L$_1$ cells by insulin and phorbol ester. Proc Natl Acad Sci USA 83: 4369–4373

Tamaoki T, Nomoto H, Takahashi I, Kato Y, Norimoto M, Tomita F (1986) Staurosporine a potent inhibitor of phospholipid/Ca^{++}-dependent protein kinase. Biochem Biophys Res Commun 135: 397–402

Thomas G, Siegmann M, Gordon J (1979) Multiple phosphorylation of ribosomal protein S6 during transition of quiescent 3T3 cells into early G1 and cellular compartimentalization of the phosphate donor. Proc Natl Acad Sci USA 76: 3952–3956

Wyss R, Fabbro D, Takahashi A, Eppenberger U (1987) Epidermal growth factor receptors and phorbol ester receptors in human breast cancer biopsies. Anticancer Res 7: 721–728

Expression of the c-erbB-2 Proto-Oncogene Protein in Human Breast Cancer

W. J. Gullick

ICRF Oncology Group, Hammersmith Hospital, 3rd Floor, MRC Cyclotron Building, Du Cane Road, London W12 OHS, Great Britain

Introduction

Analysis of the structure and expression of the human c-*erb*B-2 gene in normal and malignant cells has been stimulated by the discovery that the equivalent gene in rats, called *neu*, can be converted by mutation to a dominantly acting oncogene (Bargmann et al. 1986). Treatment of pregnant rats with the chemical carcinogen ethylnitrosourea (ENU) leads to the development of tumours of the central nervous system in the offspring. Despite the instability of the carcinogen, which has a half-life of about 5 min in vivo, the tumours appear with a long latency of about 200 days (Lantos 1986). In order to analyse the nature of the putative mutation caused by the alkylating agent ENU, DNA was prepared from a cell line derived from a rat brain tumour and transfected onto NIH-3T3 indicator cells. This assay revealed the presence of an activated DNA sequence that caused the recipient cells to be transformed to a malignant phenotype. Subsequent experiments showed that this was a gene related in structure to that encoding the epidermal growth factor (EGF) receptor (Coussens et al. 1985; Yamamoto 1986). Because of its derivation from a tumour classified as a neuroblastoma, the transforming oncogene was named onc-*neu*.

Comparison of the structure of the normal cellular rat gene, called c-*neu*, with the oncogene onc-*neu* revealed that both the predicted proteins consisted of 1260 amino acids. Only a single amino acid difference was present in the protein encoded by the onc-*neu* gene as a consequence of a single-base (T→A) transversion mutation. This same mutation was found in three more, independently derived, ENU-induced rat brain tumours suggesting either a very localised mutational event or, more likely, that a mutation at this codon was highly transforming and thus strongly selected in the assay (Bargmann et al. 1986). Interestingly, the level of expression of the mutant protein encoded by the onc-*neu* gene both in the original tumour cells and in the primary transfectant cells was quite low, essentially equivalent to that found on many normal cell types (Schechter et al. 1985).

The mechanism by which this mutation leads to transformation is not presently known, but the structural and perhaps functional relationship of the *neu* protein to the EGF receptor is provoking. The EGF receptor is a single polypeptide transmembrane glycoprotein of approximately 170000 mol wt. About half of the protein backbone of the receptor is present on the external surface of the plasma cell membrane and the remainder, linked by a transmembrane spanning sequence, is inside the cell cytoplasm. The external ligand-binding domain of the EGF receptor is heavily glycosylated, such that about 60% of the receptor structure on the outer surface of the cell membrane is composed of sugars. The internal domain consists of two parts, one adjacent to the transmembrane region which encodes the enzyme activity of protein tyrosine kinase, and a c-terminal region called the autophosphorylation site domain which, as its names suggests, can become chemically modified by the autocatalysed addition of phosphate. The rate of catalysis of the kinase domain is increased by the binding of EGF to the external domain, and it is presently hypothesised that this represents the mechanism by which information is transduced across the cell membrane (Gullick and Waterfield 1987).

Comparison of the protein encoded by the human gene equivalent to rat c-*neu*, called c-*erb*B-2, with the structure of the EGF receptor shows that the two molecules are organised in very similar ways. The c-*erb*B-2 protein is also a transmembrane protein, glycosylated on its extra-cellular domain, which is identical with the EGF receptor at 43% of its amino acid residues in this region. Strikingly, the double motif of clustered cysteine residues present in the EGF receptor is absolutely conserved in the c-*erb*B-2 protein, suggesting that they may also be similar in conformation. Whereas the transmembrane domains of the two molecules are essentially unrelated, the tyrosine kinase domains are 82% identical in sequence, indicating a possible conservation of function. Indeed, recently the *neu* and c-*erb*B-2 proteins have both been shown to possess protein tyrosine kinase activity. The c-terminal region of the c-*erb*B-2 protein contains about 40 amino acids not present in the EGF receptor, followed by a more conserved sequence, including each of the three tyrosine residues known to be sites of autophosphorylation in the EGF receptor. Thus, the two proteins are clearly distinct but contain related sequences and structural motifs, suggesting that they may have evolved from a common ancestral gene and that they might perform related functions involved in growth regulation (Coussens et al. 1985; Yamamoto et al. 1986).

The point mutation that has occurred in the onc-*neu* gene is about five amino acids inside the extracellular surface of the plasma membrane in the transmembrane spanning domain of the molecule (Bargmann et al. 1986). One possible mechanism by which this mutation converts the c-*neu* protein to an oncogene is that it leads to a permanent activation of the function of the molecule. If the c-*erb*B-2 protein is involved in the control of cell growth, this might provide a stimulus for self-renewal and consequent uncontrolled cell proliferation.

Although mutation can convert several proto-oncogenes into transforming oncogenes, other mechanisms of activation also exist. One such common mechanism which can be produced experimentally is overexpression of the un-mutated normal proto-oncogene, either by introducing many copies of the gene into cells, or by increasing the rate of transcription of the gene into mRNA. Recently, it has been shown that overexpression of the normal c-*erb*B-2 gene in NIH-3T3 cells leads to their conversion to a malignant phenotype (Di Fiore et al. 1987). However, quite high levels of expression were required for this dominant effect, since moderately elevated expression was not overtly transforming.

Thus, the c-*erb*B-2 gene encodes a molecule, related in structure to a growth factor receptor, which possesses protein tyrosine kinase activity. No ligand has been found so far which specifically interacts with the c-*neu* or c-*erb*B-2 protein, and it has thus not yet been shown that the tyrosine kinase activity of the molecules can be activated. Experiments are, however, in progress in several laboratories to investigate whether such a molecule exists and if so, what its properties are. It is apparent, however, that point mutations in the rat *neu* gene or overexpression of the human c-*erb*B-2 gene can transform cells. These interesting findings have stimulated analyses of the c-*erb*B-2 gene and its protein product in normal and transformed human cells in culture and in tissues and tumour biopsies.

Amplification of the c-*erb*B-2 Gene in Primary Breast Carcinomas

Mammalian somatic cells normally each contain two copies of any gene, one on each member of a pair of chromosomes (the exceptions to this are of course the X and Y chromosomes). Examples of additional gene copies in cells have, however, been demonstrated in two abnormal situations. Firstly, cells or tissues exposed to certain cytotoxic drugs such as methotrexate amplify genes encoding proteins capable of detoxifying the drug, thus increasing the levels of these proteins and protecting themselves from its harmful effects (Stark and Wahl 1984). This type of drug treatment provides a negative selective pressure for cells that do not increase the level of such proteins in that they are killed or damaged by the drug. Secondly, certain genes have been found to be amplified in tumour cells but not in adjacent surrounding normal tissues (Bishop 1987). This unusual event suggests that the proteins encoded by such genes may be involved in some way with the transformation process, either as an instigator or sustainer of the transformed state or as a secondary consequence or adaptation to transformation. It is, of course, also possible that they are irrelevant to this process and are simply a result of disregulation of the tumour cell genome. Evidence is emerging, however, to support the involvement of amplified genes in instigating and sustaining transformation, thereby imposing a positive selective pressure for tumour cell proliferation. Several oncogenes which have been identified in transforming retroviruses or by transfection assays have been found to be amplified in human tumor cell lines and biopsies. In other instances, such as with the c-*erb*B-2 gene, experimental overexpression leads to cell transformation.

Over the last 1 or 2 years, several studies have shown that the c-*erb*B-2 gene has become amplified in a variety of spontaneous human primary tumours. So far, amplification has been found only in adenocarcinomas, notably of the breast (King et al. 1985; Slamon et al. 1987; van de Vijver et al. 1987; Venter et al. 1987; Yokota et al. 1986) and stomach (Fukushige et al. 1986), but also single examples have been reported of amplification in a kidney tumour (Yokota et al. 1986), salivary gland tumour (Semba et al. 1985), and a colonic adenocarcinoma (Meltzer et al. 1987). No examples have been seen in sarcomas, squamous cell tumours or leukaemias, although to date limited numbers of tumours have been examined (for a review see Gullick and Venter, in press). The tumour type most intensively studied so far has been adenocarcinoma of the breast, where of nearly 400 tumours examined by Southern blotting, 25% contained additional copies of the c-*erb*B-2 gene (Gullick and Venter, 1988). In comparison with other oncogene abnormalities, this frequency and specificity of occurrence is remarkably high. The extent of gene amplification observed varies between about 2- and 20-fold, although contributions of normal cell DNA and possible heterogeneity of amplification makes this a minimum estimate. It is also possible that local gene amplification may occur in a minority of tumour cells which could not be observed by Southern blot analysis. So far, no study has reported whether amplification occurs in intraductal tumours or metastases present in lymph nodes, although as discussed below c-erbB-2 protein overexpression clearly does occur in these situations.

In the first paper describing the frequent occurrence of c-erbB-2 gene amplification in breast carcinomas (Slamon et al. 1987), the authors suggested that the presence of greater than five-fold amplification in a tumour could be statistically correlated with patients experiencing a short time to relapse and death. The amplification status of this gene was thus suggested to be a useful prognostic indicator in breast cancer. In order to examine this proposition more fully, it was apparent that since this level of amplification was observed in only about 10% of the specimens examined (Gullick and Venter, 1988), many more examples were needed in which both gene status and patient records were available. Secondly, although gene amplification was frequently observed, other mechanisms might effect a high level of c-erbB-2 protein expression leading to the same influence on tumour phenotype. This has certainly been the experience with the overexpression of the EGF receptor in human tumours, where high levels of expression have been found more commonly without than with gene amplification (Gullick and Venter, in press). The solution to these problems has been the development of antibodies capable of recognising the c-erbB-2 protein expressed in formalin-fixed paraffin-embedded tumour biopsies. Such archival material is available together with patient records in great numbers, facilitating this analysis.

Elevated Expression of the c-erbB-2 Protein in Breast Carcinomas

Immunohistological staining of normal and transformed tissues has begun to reveal the normal distribution of the c-erbB-2 protein and its frequency of overexpression in tumours. Initially, it was shown that the protein was expressed in normal epithelial cells of oral mucosa and ureter and regions of the kidney (Gullick et al. 1987). As yet, however, no systematic study of normal tissues has been reported, although it is certainly warranted. Only one report has so far appeared in which the level of expression of the c-erbB-2 protein was examined in human tumour biopsies (Venter et al. 1987), although many more are anticipated. This work demonstrated that in a series of human breast tumours there was a concomitant occurrence of c-erbB-2 gene amplification and overexpression of the protein. Subsequently, this observation has been confirmed using paraffin-embedded tissue from the same series of tumours (Gusterson et al. 1987). Several studies are now underway using these characterised reagents or other similar antibodies to examine whether c-erbB-2 protein overexpression is of prognostic value.

It is interesting that overexpression of the protein has been frequently observed in intraductal tumours and, in cases where lymph node metastases are available, that these stain similarly to the primary tumour. These observations suggest that overexpression of the protein, perhaps, but not necessarily as a consequence of gene amplification, is a relatively early event in the tumour's aetiology. This may be helpful in that if overexpression does indicate aggressive tumour behaviour, the marker is expressed at an early stage.

Finally, overexpression of any cell surface molecule on tumours as compared with normal tissues provides the opportunity for exploiting this as a target for tumour imaging or selective therapeutic cytotoxicity. A prerequisite for this approach, however, is a clear understanding of the normal distribution and level of expression of the molecule which is not yet available.

Unlike the random overexpression of any cell surface marker, it is quite conceivable that the c-erbB-2 protein is directly involved in instigating and sustaining the transformed phenotype, perhaps by expressing a growth-promoting stimulus. Thus, methods of selectively decreasing its level of expression (Drebin et al. 1986) or reducing its functional activity might temporarily aid in repressing tumour growth. This must be a limited objective, however, since there are no methods available to repair the genetic damage present in the tumour cells. Nonetheless, should it be possible to reduce the growth rate of the tumour, this combined with appropriate radiotherapy and chemotherapy and stimulation of the natural host defence systems may be of practical usefulness in therapy.

Summary

The discovery of a dominantly transforming oncogene in ENU-induced rat CNS tumours has revealed in rats and man a gene highly related to the EGF receptor. The gene may be activated experimentally by mutation or overexpression such that its expression can convert immortalised but non-tumourigenic rat fibroblasts to a tumourigenic state. The mechanism by which this activation occurs is not known, nor is it known whether the molecule is itself a growth factor receptor. It is hypothesised, however, that in the light of its similarity to the EGF receptor it may be involved in growth regulation and that activation may occur by producing an aberrant growth control signal. The gene has been found to be amplified frequently and the protein it encodes overexpressed in a variety of human adenocarcinomas. Investigations are underway to attempt to reveal its role in these tumours and to assess its possible value as an indicator of tumour behaviour. Overexpression of the protein provides a target for tumour imaging and therapy.

References

Bargmann CI, Hung M-C, Weinberg RA (1986) Multiple independent activations of the *neu* oncogene by a point mutation altering the transmembrane domain of p 185. Cell 45: 649–657

Bishop JM (1987) The molecular genetics of cancer. Science 235: 305–311

Coussens L, Yang-Feng TL, Liao Y-C, Chen E, Gray A, McGrath J, Seeberg PH, Libermann TA, Schlessinger J, Francke U, Levinson A, Ullrich A (1985) Tyrosine kinase receptor with extensive homology to EGF receptor shares chromosomal location with neu oncogene. Science 230: 1132–1139

Di Fiore PP, Pierce JH, Kraus MH, Segatto O, King CR, Aaronson SA (1987) *erb*B-2 is a potent oncogene when overexpressed in NIH/3T3 cells. Science 237: 178–182

Drebin JA, Link VC, Weinberg RA, Greene MI (1986) Inhibition of tumor growth by a monoclonal antibody reactive with an oncogene-encoded tumor antigen. Proc Natl Acad Sci USA 83: 9129–9133

Fukushige S-I, Matsubara K-I, Yoshida M, Sasaki M, Suzuki T, Semba K, Toyoshima K, Yamamoto T (1986) Localisation of a novel v-*erb*B-related gene, c-*erb*B-2, on human chromosome 17 and its amplification in a gastric cancer cell line. Mol Cell Biol 6: 955–958

Gullick WJ, Venter DJ (1988) The c-*erb*B-2 gene and its expression in human cancers. In: Sikora K, Waxman J (eds) The molecular biology of cancer. Blackwells, Oxford pp 38–53

Gullick WJ, Waterfield MD (1987) Epidermal growth factor and its receptor. In: Strosberg AD (ed) The molecular biology of receptors. Ellis Horwood, Chichester, pp 15–35

Gullick WJ, Berger MS, Bennett PLP, Rothbard JB, Waterfield MD (1987) Expression of the c-*erb*B-2 protein in normal and transformed cells. Int J Cancer 40: 246–254

Gusterson BA, Gullick WJ, Venter DJ, Powles TJ, Elliott C, Ashley S, Tidy A, Harrison S (1987) Immunohistochemical localization of c-*erb*B-2 in human breast carcinomas. Mol Cell Probes 1: 383–391

King CR, Kraus MH, Aaronson SA (1985) Amplification of a novel v-*erb*B-related gene in a human mammary carcinoma. Science 229: 974–976

Lantos PL (1986) Development of nitrosourea-induced brain tumours – with a special note on changes occurring during latency. Fd Chem Toxic 24: 121–127

Meltzer SJ, Ahnen DJ, Battifora H, Yokota J, Cline MJ (1987) Proto-oncogene abnormalities in colon cancers and adenomatous polyps. Gastroenterology 92: 1174–1180

Schechter AL, Hung M-C, Vaidyanathan L, Weinberg RA, Yang-Feng TL, Francke U, Ullrich A, Coussens L (1985) The neu gene: An erbB-homologous gene distinct from and unlinked to the gene encoding the EGF receptor. Science 229: 976–978

Semba K, Kamata N, Toyoshima K, Yamamoto T (1985) A v-*erb*B related proto-oncogene, c-*erb*B-2, is distinct from the c-*erb*B-1/epidermal growth factor-receptor gene and is amplified in a human salivary gland adenocarcinoma. Proc Natl Acad Sci USA 82: 6497–6501

Slamon DJ, Clark GM, Wong SG, Levin WJ, Ullrich A, McGuire WL (1987) Human breast cancer: correlation of relapse and survival with amplification of the HER-2/neu oncogene. Science 235: 177–182

Stark GR, Wahl GM (1984) Gene amplification. Ann Rev Biochem 53: 447–491

Van de Vijver M, van de Bersselaar R, Devilee P, Cornelisse C, Peterse J, Nusse R (1987) Amplification of the neu (c-*erb*B-2) oncogene in human mammary tumors is relatively frequent and is often accompanied by amplification of the linked c-*erb*A oncogene. Mol Cell Biol 7: 2019–2023

Venter DJ, Tuzi NL, Kumar S, Gullick WJ (1987) Overexpression of the c-*erb*B-2 oncoprotein in human breast carcinomas: Immunohistological assessment correlates with gene amplification. Lancet ii: 69–72

Yamomoto T, Ikawa S, Akiyama T, Semba K, Nomura N, Miyajima N, Saito T, Toyoshima K (1986) Similarity of protein encoded by the human c-*erb*B-2 gene to epidermal growth factor receptor. Nature 319: 230–234

Yokota J, Yamamoto T, Toyoshima K, Terada M, Sugimura T, Battifora H, Chine MJ (1986) Amplification of c-*erb*B-2 oncogene in human adenocarcinomas in vivo. Lancet i: 765–766

Modulation by Estrogen and Growth Factors of Transforming Growth Factor-Alpha and Epidermal Growth Factor Receptor Expression in Normal and Malignant Human Mammary Epithelial Cells

D. S. Salomon[1], W. R. Kidwell[1], N. Kim[1], F. Ciardiello[1], S. E. Bates[2], E. Valverius[2], M. E. Lippman[2], R. B. Dickson[2], and M. Stampfer[3]

[1] Laboratory of Tumor Immunology and Biology, National Cancer Institute, National Institutes of Health, Bethesda, MD 20892, USA
[2] Medicine Branch, National Cancer Institutes, National Institutes of Health, Bethesda, MD 20892, USA
[3] Lawrence Berkeley Laboratory. University of California, Berkeley, CA 94720, USA

Introduction

A number of well-characterized growth factors, such as epidermal growth factor (EGF) and the insulin-like growth factors (IGFs), can stimulate the proliferation and modify the differentiation of normal and malignant rodent and human mammary epithelial cells (Salomon et al. 1986 a, c). For example, EGF or transforming growth factor-alpha (TGFα) can stimulate the lobulo-alveolar development of mouse mammary glands in organ culture or in vivo (Tonelli and Soroff 1980; Okamoto and Oka 1984; Vonderhaar 1987). In addition, EGF may perform a physiological role in the development of the mouse mammary gland during pregnancy and lactation and in the spontaneous formation of mammary tumors in mice (Okamoto and Oka 1984; Oka et al. 1987; Tsutsumi et al. 1987). Several of these growth factors, such as IGF-I, platelet-derived growth factor (PDGF), TGFα, and TGFβ, have been found in the conditioned medium (CM) from several human breast cancer cell lines (Salomon et al. 1984; Dickson et al. 1986; Huff et al. 1986; Bronzert et al. 1987; Knabbe et al. 1987; Peres et al. 1987). The production of TGFα, IGF-I, and TGFβ can be modulated by estrogens or anti-estrogens, suggesting that the growth-promoting effects of estrogen may be mediated in part by TGFα and/or IGF-I and that the growth-inhibitory effects of anti-estrogen may be mediated by TGFβ (Dickson et al. 1985; Perroteau et al. 1986; Knabbe et al. 1987; Liu et al. 1987; Peres et al. 1987; Huff et al. 1988). However, it is still unclear whether these or other growth factors are present in mammary tumor cells in vivo and, if so, whether they are involved in the etiology of tumor development and progression. Likewise, there is little information on the distribution and level of expression of similar growth factors in normal mammary epithelial cells at specific times during the development of the mammary gland.

We have been studying the function and expression of a class of growth factors, transforming growth factors (TGFs), that has been circumstantially implicated in controlling the growth of a variety of rodent and human tumor cells in an autocrine manner (Roberts and Sporn 1985; Derynck 1986). Specifically, we have focused our attention on TGFα, since this growth factor is structurally and functionally related to EGF and binds to and operates through the EGF receptor (EGFR) (Derynck 1986). TGFα (M_r 5400) is a 50-amino-acid peptide, that is a potent mitogen for fibroblasts and epithelial cells and cooperates with TGFβ to reversibly confer upon normal nontransformed cells several properties that are associated with the transformed phenotype, namely anchorage-independent growth (AIG) in semi-solid medium and a loss of anchorage-dependent, contact inhibition of growth. The genes for mouse, rat, and human TGFα have been cloned, and the size of the messenger ribonucleic acid (mRNA), approximately 4.8 kb, indicates that TGFα of low molecular weight is derived from a 160-amino-acid-membrane-associated precursor specie(s) (Bringman et al. 1987; Gentry et al. 1987). Larger biologically and immunologically active precursor-like molecules have been identified in several rodent and human tumor cell lines and from human urine and milk (Ignotz et al. 1986; Zwiebel et al. 1986; Stromberg et al. 1987).

TGFα in Human Breast Cancer Cell Lines

TGFα, which is capable of competing with EGF in a EGF radioreceptor assay (RRA) and able to induce the AIG of normal rat kidney (NRK) cells in soft agar in the presence of exogenous TGFβ, has been detected in the crude or partially purified acid-ethanol extracts prepared from rodent and human mammary tumors and from the CM obtained from the human breast cancer cell lines MCF-7, T47-D, ZR-75-1, and MDA-MB-231 (Salomon et al. 1984; Dickson et al. 1985, 1986; Perroteau et al. 1986). In the case of MCF-7 and MDA-MB-231 cells, the TGFα species that are secreted into the CM are 30000 and 6000 M_r proteins, which probably represents a precursor, and the peptide of low molecular weight (Dickson et al. 1986). A comparable 30000-M_r protein could also be detected in the CM after biosynthetic labeling of MCF-7 cells with [^{35}S]cysteine followed by immunoprecipitation of the CM with a polyclonal goat anti-human TGFα antibody (Bates et al. 1988). The radiolabeled 30000-M_r protein could be eliminated by preincubation of the TGFα antibody with an excess of unlabeled recombinant TGFα of low molecular weight. The 6000- and 30000-M_r TGFα proteins were biologically active in an EGF RRA and in promoting the AIG of NRK cells in soft agar.

The production of TGFα may be functionally significant for the growth of a subset of human breast cancer cells. For example, incubation of MCF-7 cells with a polyclonal rabbit anti-human TGFα-neutralizing antibody could produce a 60% inhibition in the AIG of MCF-7 cells in soft agar (Bates et al. 1988). This effect was not evident with pre-immune rabbit serum or with rabbit anti-human TGFα antibody that had been preabsorbed with an excess of recombinant human TGFα. In addition, incubation of MCF-7 cells with a mouse monoclonal anti-human EGFR-blocking antibody could produce a 40%–50% inhibition in the estrogen-induced growth of MCF-7 cells in monolayer culture. These results suggest that, by either neutralizing TGFα or by blocking the receptor with which TGFα interacts, mammary tumor cell growth can be reduced.

The results obtained with the EGF RRA or with the NRK soft agar bioassay did not unequivocally demonstrate that the activity elaborated by the human breast cancer cell lines was due to authentic TGFα and not due to the presence of

EGF. However, immunoreactive human EGF could not be detected in the CM from the breast cancer cell lines (Perroteau et al. 1986). More importantly, using a highly sensitive and specific radioimmunoassay (RIA) for TGFα with an antibody that does not cross-react with mouse or human EGF, authentic immunoreactive TGFα could be detected and quantitated in the CM from the four human breast cancer cell lines, in tissue extracts prepared from normal, benign, and malignant breast biopsies, and in pleural effusions and urine from breast cancer patients (Hanauske et al. 1988; Perroteau et al. 1986; Stromberg et al. 1987). The levels of TGFα in the CM from the breast cancer cell lines ranged from 35 to 0.5 ng/10^8 cells. The MDA-MB-231 cells had higher levels of biologically active and immunoreactive TGFα than the other three breast cancer cell lines (Dickson et al. 1985, 1986; Perroteau et al. 1986).

Modulation of TGFα Production by Estrogens

Treatment of the estrogen-responsive MCF-7 and ZR-75-1 breast cancer cell lines with 17β-estradiol (10^{-8} M) for 48 h results in a 3- to 5-fold increase in the CM levels of TGFα compared with control cultures (Dickson et al. 1985, 1986; Perroteau et al. 1986). These results were confirmed by Northern blot analysis by hybridization of a full-length, nick-translated, labeled human TGFα 850-bp cDNA

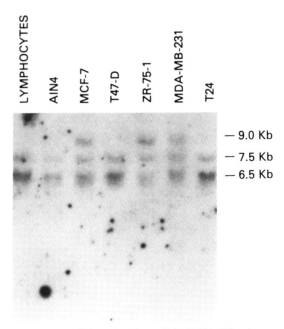

Fig. 1. Southern blot analysis of the TGFα gene. High molecular weight DNA (10 µg) was digested with *Bam*HI before being fractionated on 0.8% agarose gels, transferred to nitrocellulose membranes, and hybridized and washed under highly stringent conditions. DNA was hybridized to a TGFα, cDNA-cloned insert, pTGF-CI that was nick-translated with ^{32}P. *T24,* human bladder carcinoma cell line; for explanation of remaining abbreviations, see text

insert to poly(A)$^+$ RNA isolated from the breast cancer cell lines and from MCF-7 cells grown in nude mice as tumor xenografts (Salomon et al. 1986b; Bates et al. 1988). A major 4.8-kb and a minor 1.6-kb TGFα mRNA species were detected in all four of the breast cancer cell lines (Derynck et al. 1987; Bates et al. 1988). The relative basal levels of TGFα mRNA expression correlated reasonable well with the amount of immunoreactive TGFα that could be detected in the CM from these cells. Moreover, estrogen treatment of MCF-7 cells produced a 2- to 3-fold increase in TGFα mRNA expression within 6 h; these cells exhibited a dose-dependent increase in the levels of TGFα mRNA after 48 h of treatment. Maximum induction of TGFα mRNA expression occurred at between 10^{-9} and 10^{-8} M estradiol. A similar estrogen-dependent response in TGFα mRNA expression could be demonstrated in vivo in the growth of MCF-7 xenografts in nude mice and in the growth of a subset of carcinogen-induced, estrogen-dependent differentiated rat mammary adenocarcinomas (Liu et al. 1987; Bates et al. 1988). Withdrawal of the exogenous estrogen pellets from MCF-7 tumor-bearing nude mice resulted in a 2- to 3-fold decrease in TGFα mRNA expression in the tumors within 24-48 h, preceding any change in tumor growth rate. Ovariectomy produced a 90% reduction within 6 h of TGFα mRNA levels in primary carcinogen-induced rat mammary tumors. Figure 1 shows that according to Southern analysis of genomic DNA digested with *Bam*HI and hybridized to the nick-translated, labeled TGFα cDNA probe, there was no evidence for amplification or major rearrangements of the TGFα gene in any of the breast cancer cell lines. This was shown as compared with the restriction endonuclease pattern of DNA isolated from normal human peripheral blood lymphocytes or from A1N4 cells, a subline of the immortalized normal human mammary epithelial cell line (184A1N4) developed by Stampfer and Bartley (1985).

TGFα in Primary Human Breast Tumors

TGFα is not restricted to human breast cancer cell lines, since it can be detected in primary human breast tumors (Perroteau et al. 1986; Macias et al. 1987). For example, in acid extracts prepared from normal breast tissue, a benign fibrocystic lesion, two fibroadenomas, and 22 primary infiltrating ductal breast carcinomas, immunoreactive TGFα concentrations were found to range from 1.5 to 6.0 ng/mg protein (Perroteau et al. 1986). Approximately 50% of the breast carcinomas possessed TGFα levels greater than 2.5 ng/mg protein, values exceeding those found in the normal or benign breast tissues. Fifteen infiltrating ductal carcinomas were also examined for the presence of TGFα mRNA after Northern blot hybridization of the tumor poly(A)$^+$ RNA with a labeled 400-bp human TGFα antisense riboprobe (Salomon et al. 1986b). Of these tumors 53% (8 of 15) were found to contain a 4.8-kb TGFα mRNA species. Within this group of tumors, 75% (6 of 8) of the tumors were estrogen receptor (ER) positive/progesterone receptor (PgR) positive, while the remaining 25% (2 of 8) were ER negative/PgR negative. In the TGFα mRNA-negative tumor group (7 of 15), 71% (5 of 7) were ER negative/PgR negative. A second group of 36 primary human breast tumors was also examined for TGFα mRNA expression (Bates et al. 1988).

In approximately 72% (26 of 36) of this group of tumors, TGFα mRNA could be detected. However, in this group of tumors, no correlation could be discerned between ER and/or PgR status and TGFα mRNA expression, since equal numbers of ER-positive and ER-negative tumors were present in the 26 tumors that were positive for TGFα mRNA. We are presently conducting a more extensive investigation to determine whether there is any correlation between TGFα production or TGFα mRNA expression and tumor size, axillary lymph node involvement, stage, and EGF receptor expression.

TGFα Production by Normal Human Mammary Epithelial Cells and Modulation by Growth Factors

Expression of TGFα may not be entirely restricted to those mammary epithelial cells that are malignant. We have previously demonstrated the presence of at least three distinct TGFα species in human milk (Salomon and Kidwell, 1988; Zwiebel et al. 1986). One of these TGFα variants has been purified and has been found to be identical to the TGFα activity detectable in primary human breast tumors

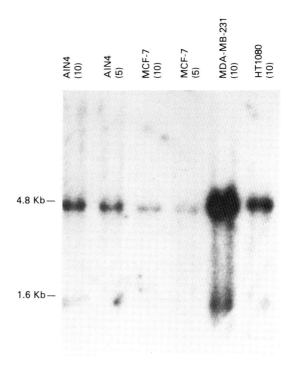

Fig. 2. Northern blot analysis of TGFα mRNA. Poly(A)⁺ RNA was isolated from A1N4 cells, MCF-7 and MDA-MB-231 human breast cancer cells, or from the HT-1080 human fibrosarcoma cell line (positive control). The RNA was denatured and 5 or 10 μg of RNA were fractionated on 1% denaturing agarose gels and transferred to nitrocellulose. RNA was hybridized to the nick-translated TGFα cDNA probe under stringent conditions and washed with 0.1 × standard saline citrate

(Zwiebel et al. 1986). These results suggest that normal mammary epithelial cells may have the capacity to synthesize and secrete TGFα. This may be the case, as we have recently demonstrated that cultures of proliferating normal human mammary epithelial cells, which were established from organoids obtained from reductive mammaplasties, secrete biologically active and immunoreactive TGFα. These cells secrete TGFα at levels that are comparable to those observed in the CM from the MCF-7 and MDA-MB-231 breast cancer cell lines and express a 4.8-kb TGFα mRNA (Perroteau et al. 1989; Valverius et al. 1989). In addition, A1N4 cells, an immortalized human mammary epithelial cell line, also secrete TGFα at levels ranging from 30 to 40 ng/10^8 cells (Salomon and Kidwell, 1988). Figure 2 is a Northern blot that demonstrates the presence of a 4.8-kb TGFα mRNA in proliferating A1N4 cells at levels that exceed those observed in the MCF-7 breast cancer cell line. A1N4 cells are unique in that they exhibit a requirement for exogenous EGF for growth in monolayer cultures in Improved Minimum Eagle's medium (IMEM) in low concentrations of fetal calf serum (0.5%) in the presence of insulin (10 µg/ml), transferin (10 µg/ml), and hydrocortisone (0.5 µg/ml). In the absence of added EGF or TGFα, A1N4 cells fail to proliferate and remain quiescent. Figure 3 demonstrates that the addition of either recombinant human EGF or recombinant human TGFα to A1N4 cells produces a 3- to 5-fold increase in cell growth between 5 and 10 ng/ml. Addition of porcine TGFβ has no effect on cell growth in the absence of either EGF or TGFα. However, TGFβ can synergistically

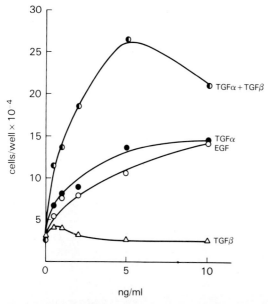

Fig. 3. Effect of human EGF, human TGFα, and porcine TGFβ on the anchorage-dependent growth of A1N4 cells. A1N4 cells (2.5×10^4) were seeded in IMEM medium containing 0.5% fetal calf serum, insulin and transferrin (10 µg/ml each), and hydrocortisone (0.5 µg/ml) in the absence or presence of different concentrations of EGF (○——○), TGFα (●——●), TGFβ (△——△), or TGFα plus TGFβ (2 ng/ml, ◐——◐). Cells were cultured for 4 days before counting

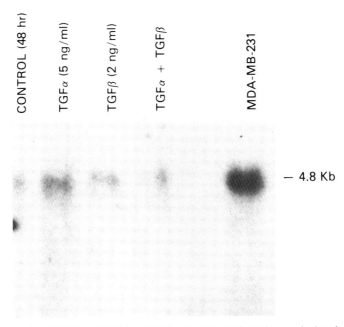

CONTROL (48 hr)   TGFα (5 ng/ml)   TGFβ (2 ng/ml)   TGFα + TGFβ   MDA-MB-231

— 4.8 Kb

Fig. 4. Northern blot analysis of TGFα mRNA in A1N4 cells. Poly(A)$^+$ RNA was isolated from MDA-MB-231 breast cancer cells or from A1N4 cells that had been grown in the absence (control) or presence of TGFα (5 ng/ml), TGFβ (2 ng/ml), or TGFα (5 ng/ml) plus TGFβ (2 ng/ml) for 48 h. Poly(A)$^+$ RNA (5 µg) was electrophoresed and hybridized to the labeled TGFα cDNA probe as described in the legend of Fig. 2

enhance the growth-promoting effects of either TGFα or EGF (data not shown). Interestingly, the level of endogenous TGFα that is secreted into the CM from quiescent A1N4 cells (2–4 ng/10^8 cells) is significantly lower than the CM levels of TGFα obtained from A1N4 cells that are rapidly proliferating in the presence of exogenous EGF (approx. 40 ng/10^8 cells). These results were confirmed by Northern blot analysis (Fig. 4). Following a 48-h exposure of A1N4 cells to TGFα (5 ng/ml) but not to TGFβ (2 ng/ml), TGFα mRNA expression was increased 2- to 3-fold over TGFα mRNA levels in A1N4 cells grown in the absence of exogenous TGFα. The results suggest that increased production of TGFα in normal mammary epithelial cells may occur during rapid cell growth, and that the exogenous levels of TGFα or EGF, which both interact through the EGFR, might control the expression of TGFα through a positive feedback loop. A similar result has recently been documented for TGFα expression in primary cultures of human keratinocytes (Coffey et al. 1987).

Expression of EGF Receptors in A1N4 Human Mammary Epithelial Cells

A1N4 cells are also unusual because they express high levels of EGFRs (Valverius et al. 1989). Figure 5 illustrates the specific binding of ^{125}I-labeled EGF at various concentrations to A1N4 cells at 22 °C. Scatchard analysis of the binding curve in-

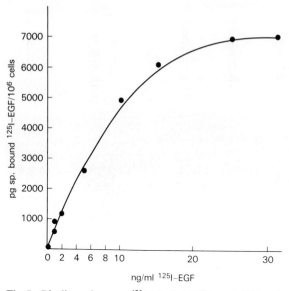

Fig. 5. Binding of mouse ^{125}I-labeled EGF to A1N4 cells. Specific binding was determined at 22 °C with different concentrations of ^{125}I-labeled EGF. Nonspecific binding was corrected by the inclusion of 500 ng/ml of unlabeled mouse EGF in parallel wells

dicates that there are approximately 1.8×10^6 binding sites per cell and at least two different classes of receptor sites since a curvilinear Scatchard plot was observed. Receptor levels ranged from 0.5 to 2×10^6 sites/cell in several different experiments (Valverius et al. 1989). The high-affinity Kd of EGFRs on the A1N4 cells was calculated to be approximately 2.6×10^{-11} M, while the low-affinity Kd was 9.26×10^{-10} M. It should be noted that overexpression of EGFRs is a property that is usually associated with certain malignant epithelial cells (Merlino et al. 1984; Libermann et al. 1985; Filmus et al. 1987). However, A1N4 cells are not transformed because they fail to grow in soft agar and because they are not tumorigenic in nude mice (Stampfer and Bartley 1984). Increased expression of EGFRs may confer a selective growth advantage on cells under EGF-limiting conditions (Filmus et al. 1987). This may account for the enhanced sensitivity of A1N4 cells to the growth-promoting effects of EGF. In contrast to other tumor cells, such as A-431 epidermoid carcinoma cells or the MDA-MB-468 breast cancer cells, which both possess equally high numbers of EGFRs (Merlino et al. 1984; Filmus et al. 1987), EGF over a wide concentration range is not growth inhibitory to A1N4 cells.

Poly(A)$^+$ RNA from the A1N4 cells was hybridized to the nick-translated, labeled human cDNA clone, pE7, which encodes 2.4 kb of the human EGFR (Merlino et al. 1984) to determine whether the increased binding of EGF observed on the AIN4 cells was due to an overexpression of EGFR mRNA species. Figure 6 illustrates a typical Northern blot of the EGFR mRNA species detected in A1N4 cells that had been grown in the absence or presence of TGFα (5 ng/ml) and/or TGFβ (2 ng/ml) for 48 h. Distinct 10-kb and 5.8-kb EGFR mRNA species

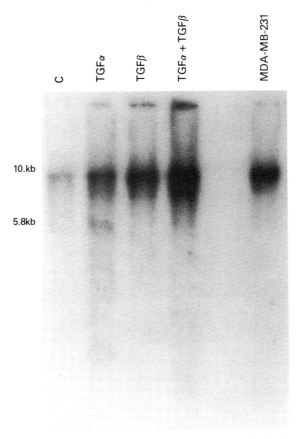

Fig. 6. Northern blot analysis of EGFR mRNA in A1N4 cells. Poly(A)⁺ RNA was isolated from MDA-MB-231 cells and from A1N4 cells grown under the conditions as described in the legend of Fig. 4. Poly(A)⁺ RNA (10 μg) was electrophoresed and hybridized to the labeled nick-translated 2.4 kb pE7 EGFR cDNA probe under stringent conditions. *C*, controls; for explanation of other abbreviations, see text

were detected in the A1N4 cells. These are similar to the EGFR mRNA species previously detected in other cell lines (Merlino et al. 1984; Libermann et al. 1985; Filmus et al. 1987). It has recently been demonstrated that EGF or TGFβ can bring about an increase in EGFR mRNA expression in several rodent and human cell lines (Clark et al. 1985; Fernandez-Pol et al. 1987). This effect may relate to the ability of EGF and/or TGFβ to regulate cell proliferation. This response may also occur in A1N4 cells, since TGFα or TGFβ is able to induce a 20- to 40-fold increase in EGFR mRNA expression, while addition of both growth factors induces a nearly 100-fold increase in EGFR mRNA levels over those in cells not treated with either growth factor.

In the majority of instances where there is an overexpression of EGFR mRNA and EGFR protein, this effect can be accounted for by an amplification and/or rearrangement of the EGFR (c-*erb B*) gene (Merlino et al. 1984; King et al. 1985;

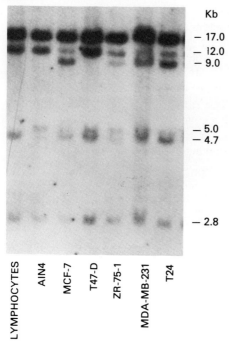

Fig. 7. Southern blot analysis of the EGFR gene. High molecular weight DNA (10 μg) was digested with *Hind* III before being fractionated on 0.8% agarose gels, transferred to nitrocellulose membranes, and hybridized to the labeled pE7 EGFR cDNA probe under highly stringent conditions

Libermann et al. 1985; Filmus et al. 1987). Figure 7 demonstrates a Southern blot of DNA samples that were obtained from A1N4 cells, the four human breast cancer cell lines, and normal human peripheral blood lymphocytes. The DNA was digested with *Hind* III prior to electrophoresis, transfer, and hybridization with the pE7 nick-translated EGFR cDNA probe. No evidence for amplification or gross rearrangements of the EGFR gene was observed in the A1N4 cells or in the human breast cancer cell-lines as compared with the EGFR gene in peripheral blood lymphocytes. These results are consistent with the data demonstrating that overexpression of EGFRs in A1N4 cells occurs at the level of transcription and that the enhanced growth sensitivity of these cells to either exogenous EGF or TGFα is due in part to the cells' increased expression of the EGFR gene and to the enhanced production of endogenous TGFα, both of which can be up-regulated by those two growth factors.

Conclusions

In summary, the results demonstrate first that TGFα expression, secretion, and operation through the EGFR system is occurring in normal, immortalized and malignant human mammary epithelial cells. Second, the results suggest that the rate of normal and malignant mammary cell growth is probably being controlled in part by several endogenously derived growth factors such as TGFα. Finally, estrogens, along with other endogenously or systemically derived growth factors, may modulate the production of TGFα and EGFR levels in normal and malignant mammary epithelial cells. The presence of TGFα in normal mammary epithelial cells and in human milk further suggests that under certain developmental conditions the mammary gland may be producing TGFα and that TGFα could perform a function in the developing neonate. It is important to emphasize that normal and malignant mammary epithelial cells are elaborating several distinct growth factors (Salomon et al. 1986a, 1986c). The concerted action of these multiple factors may be necessary for regulating the growth of these cells through an autocrine mechanism and/or stimulating the proliferation of surrounding stromal or endothelial cells in a paracrine fashion and thereby contributing to the processes of desmoplasia and angiogenesis. Furthermore, the recent demonstration that overexpression of a transfected TGFα gene in normal recipient rodent fibroblasts is able to convert these cells into transformed cells supports a role for TGFα in the etiology of tumor formation (Rosenthal et al. 1986).

References

Bates SE, Davidson NE, Valverius E, Dickson RB, Freter CE, Tam JP, Kudlow JE, Lippman ME, Salomon DS (1988) Expression of transforming growth factor alpha and its messenger ribonucleic acid in human breast cancer: its regulation by estrogen and its evidence for an autocrine role. Mol Endocrinol 2: 543–555

Bringman TS, Lindquist PB, Derynck R (1987) Different transforming growth factor-α species are derived from glycosylated and palmitoylated transmembrane precursor. Cell 48: 429–440

Bronzert DA, Pantazis P, Antoniades HN, Kasid A, Davidson N, Dickson RB, Lippman ME (1987) Synthesis and secretion of platelet-derived growth factor by human breast cancer cell lines. Proc Natl Acad Sci USA 84: 5763–5767

Clark AJL, Ishia S, Richert N, Merlino GT, Pastan I (1985) Epidermal growth factor regulates the expression of its own receptor. Proc Natl Acad Sci USA 82: 8374–8378

Coffey RJ, Derynck R, Wilcox JN, Bringman TS, Goustin AS, Moses HL, Pittelkow MR (1987) Production and auto-induction of transforming growth factor-α in human keratinocytes. Nature 328: 817–820

Derynck R (1986) Transforming growth factor-α: structure and biological activities. J Cell Biochem 32: 293–304

Derynck R, Goeddel DV, Ulrich A, Gutterman JU, Williams RD, Bringman TS, Berger WH (1987) Synthesis of messenger RNAs for transforming growth factors α and β and the epidermal growth factor receptor by human tumors. Cancer Res 47: 707–712

Dickson RB, Huff KK, Spencer EM, Lippman ME (1985) Induction of epidermal growth factor-related polypeptides by 17β-estradiol in human breast cancer cells. Endocrinology 118: 138–142

Dickson RB, Bates SE, McManaway ME, Lippman ME (1986) Characterization of estrogen responsive transforming activity in human breast cancer cell lines. Cancer Res 46: 1707–1713

Fernandez-Pol JA, Klos DJ, Hamilton PD, Talkad VD (1987) Modulation of epidermal growth factor receptor gene expression by transforming growth factor-β in a human breast carcinoma cell line. Cancer Res 47: 4260–4265

Filmus J, Trent JM, Pollak MN, Buick RN (1987) Epidermal growth factor receptor gene-amplified MDA-468 breast cancer cell line and its nonamplified variants. Mol Cell Biol 7: 251–257

Gentry LE, Twardzik DR, Lim JG, Ranchalis JE, Lee DC (1987) Expression and characterization of transforming growth factor-α precursor in transfected mammalian cells. Mol Cell Biol 7: 1585-1591

Hanauske A-R, Arteaga CL, Clark GM, Buchok J, Marshall M, Hazarika P,, Pardue RL, von Hoff DD (1988) Determination of transforming growth factor activity in effusions from cancer patients. Cancer 61: 1832-1887

Huff KK, Kaufman D, Gabbay KH, Spencer EM, Lippman ME, Dickson RB (1986) Human breast cancer cells secrete an insulin-like growth factor-I-related polypeptide. Cancer Res 46: 4613-4619

Huff KK, Knabbe C, Lindsey R, Kaufman D, Bronzert D, Lippman ME, Dickson RB (1988) Multihormonal regulation of insulin-like growth factor-I-related protein in MCF-7 human breast cancer cells. Mol Endocrinol 2: 200-208

Ignotz RA, Kelly B, Davis RJ, Massague J (1986) Biologically active precursor for transforming growth factor type α, released by retrovirally transformed cells. Proc Natl Acad Sci USA 83: 6307-6311

King CR, Kraus MH, Williams LT, Merlino GT, Pastan I, Aronson SA (1985) Human tumor cell lines with EGF receptor gene amplification in the absence of aberrant size mRNAs. Nucleic Acids Res 13: 8477-8486

Knabbe C, Lippman ME, Wakefield LM, Flanders KC, Kasid A, Derynck R, Dickson RB (1987) Evidence that transforming growth factor β is a hormonally regulated negative growth factor in human breast cancer cells. Cell 48: 417-428

Libermann TA, Nusbaum HR, Razon N, Razon R, Kris I, Lax H, Soret N, White A, Waterfield MD, Ulrich A, Schlessinger J (1985) Amplification, enhanced expression, and possible rearrangement of EGF receptor gene in primary human brain tumors of glial origin. Nature 313: 144-147

Liu SC, Sanfilippo B, Perroteau I, Derynck R, Salomon DS, Kidwell WR (1987) Expression of transforming growth factor α (TGFα) in differentiated rat mammary tumors: estrogen induction of TGFα production. Mol Endocrinol 1: 683-692

Merlino GT, Xu Y-H, Ishii S, Clark AJL, Sermba K. Toyoshima T, Yamamoto T, Pastan I (1984) Amplification and enhanced expression of the epidermal growth factor receptor gene in A-431 human carcinoma cells. Science 224: 417-419

Oka T, Kurachi H, Yoshimura M, Tsutsumi I, Cossu M, Taga M (1987) Study of the growth factors for the mammary gland: epidermal growth factor and mesenchyme-derived growth factors. Nucl Med Biol 14: 353-360

Macias A, Perez R, Hagerström T, Skooy L (1987) Identification of transforming growth factor alpha in human primary breast carcinomas. Anticancer Res 7: 1271-1276

Okamoto S, Oka T (1984) Evidence for a physiological function of epidermal growth factor: pregestational sialadenectomy of mice decreases milk production and increases offspring mortality during lactation period. Proc Natl Acad Sci USA 81: 6059-6063

Peres R, Betsholtz C, Westermark B, Heldin C-H (1987) Frequent expression of growth factors for mesenchymal cells in human mammary carcinoma cell lines. Cancer Res 47: 3425-3429

Perroteau I, Salomon DS, DeBortoli M, Kidwell W, Hazarika P, Pardue R, Dedman J, Tam J (1986) Immunological detection and quantitation of alpha transforming growth factor in human breast carcinoma cells. Breast Cancer Res Treat 7: 201-210

Roberts AB, Sporn MB (1985) Transforming growth factors. Cancer Surv 4: 684-705

Rosenthal A, Lindquist PB, Bringman TS, Goeddel DV, Derynck R (1986) Expression in rat fibroblasts of a human transforming growth factor-α cDNA results in transformation. Cell 46: 301-309

Salomon DS, Kidwell WR (1988) Tumor-associated growth factors in malignant rodent and human mammary epithelial cells. In: Lippman ME, Dickson RB (eds) Breast cancer: cellular and molecular biology, Kluwer Academic Publishers, Boston, MA, pp 361-389

Salomon DS, Zwiebel JA, Bano M, Losonczy I, Fehnel P, Kidwell WR (1984) Presence of transforming growth factors in human breast cancer cells. Cancer Res 44: 4069-4077

Salomon DS, Bano M, Kidwell WR (1986a) Polypeptide growth factors and the growth of mammary epithelial cells. In: Rich MA, Hayes JC, Papadimitrion J-T (eds) Breast cancer: origins, detection and treatment. Martinus Nijhoff, Boston, pp 42–56

Salomon DS, Kidwell WR, Liu S, Kim N, Callahan R, Theillet C, Lidereau R, Derynck R (1986b) Presence of alpha TGF mRNA in human breast cancer cell lines and in human breast carcinomas. Breast Cancer Res Treat 8: 106 (abstract no. 109)

Salomon DS, Perroteau I, Kidwell WR (1986c) Tumor-derived growth factors in rodent and human mammary carcinoma cells. In: Eppenberger U, Fabbro D, Schäfer P (eds) Endocrine therapy of breast cancer. Karger, Basel, pp 5–16. Contributions to oncology, vol 23

Stampfer MR, Bartley JC (1985) Induction of transformation and continuous cell lines from normal human mammary epithelial cells after exposure to benzo [a] pyrene. Proc Natl Acad Sci USA 82: 2394–2398

Stromberg K, Hudgins WR, Orth DN (1987) Urinary TGFs in neoplasia: immunoreactive TGF-α in the urine of patients with disseminated breast carcinoma. Biochem Biophys Res Commun 144: 1059–1068

Tonelli QJ, Soroff S (1980) Epidermal growth factor requirement for development of cultured mammary glands. Nature 285: 250–252

Tsutsumi O, Tsutsumi A, Oka T (1987) Importance of epidermal growth factor in implantation and growth of mouse mammary tumor in female nude mice. Cancer Res 47: 4651–4653

Valverius EM, Bates SE, Stampfer MR, Clark R, McCormick F, Salomon DS, Lippman ME, Dickson RB (1989) Transforming growth factor alpha production and EGF receptor expression in normal and oncogene transformed human mammary epithelial cells. Mol Endocrinol (in press)

Vonderhaar BK (1987) Local effects of EGF, α-TGF, and EGF-like growth factors on lobuloalveolar development of the mouse mammary gland in vivo. J Cell Physiol 132: 581–584

Zwiebel JA, Bano M, Nexo E, Salomon DS, Kidwell WR (1986) Partial purification of transforming growth factors from human milk. Cancer Res 46: 933–939

Epidermal Growth Factor Receptor in Human Breast Cancer

A. L. Harris

ICRF Clinical Oncology Unit, Churchill Hospital, Headington,
Oxford OX3 7LJ, Great Britain

Epidermal Growth Factor Receptor in Human Breast Cancer

The study of the epidermal growth factor (EGF) receptor in human breast cancer has been of major interest. The most widely used method of receptor identification has been a radioligand assay in which ^{125}I-labelled EGF is incubated with membranes prepared from both primary and metastatic tumours, both alone and in the presence of a large excess of unlabelled EGF, the difference in binding under these two conditions representing specific binding (for review, see Carpenter 1985). Minor differences in methodology exist between the groups who have published in this field, but some important and consistent observations can be made. High-affinity binding specific for EGF is present in 30%–50% of primary breast tumours (Sainsbury et al., 1985; Perez et al., 1984; Fitzpatrick et al., 1984; Fabbro et al., 1986), with levels of 1–120 fmol/mg receptor protein deduced usually by Scatchard analysis of binding data.

However, there is no general agreement on a clinically significant level. The three original publications all analysed oestrogen receptor levels by the dextran-coated charcoal method, and one group also analysed progesterone receptor levels (Fitzpatrick et al., 1984). Two groups arbitrarily chose a cut-off point of 1 fmol/mg membrane protein (Perez et al., 1984; Fitzpatrick et al., 1984), but in our department a higher level was used (Sainsbury et al., 1985).

Measurement of EGFr in Human Breast Cancer

It is worth describing our method in some detail because of the differing results others have found. Freshly collected tumour membranes were prepared by homogenisation in 10 mM Tris HCl/50 mM NaCl, pH 7.4, followed by centrifugation at 800 g. The supernatant was then centrifuged at 100000 g for 35 min. The pellet contained the membrane fraction. EGF was labelled by the iodogen method to a specific activity of approximately 80–130 µCi/µg. In ligand binding assays, 100-fold excess EGF was used to determine nonspecific binding. Time-course studies showed equilibration with binding sites within 60 min at 26 °C.

Scatchard analyses were carried out in two ways. Firstly, a fixed concentration of 0.3 nM EGF was used and increasing concentrations of unlabelled EGF. Alternatively, increasing concentrations of labelled EGF can be used. A direct compari-

Recent Results in Cancer Research, Vol. 113
© Springer-Verlag Berlin·Heidelberg 1989

son of the methods on the same tumours shows that the second method defines more precisely the affinity of high-affinity sites, but both give similar results for receptor density of the high-affinity sites.

In an initial screen of a tumour, we carried out a two-point assay in triplicate. Initially this used 0.6 nM labelled EGF, in order to identify particularly the high-affinity site. More recently, this has been increased to 1 nM to increase the sensitivity of the assay. The criteria used for the interpretation of these assays is crucial. An unpaired t test between the three figures for total binding and the three for nonspecific binding is performed and if the difference reaches the 95% confidence limit ($p < 0.05$), and specific binding is $> 0.25\%$ (equivalent to 10 fm/mg), then the tumour is considered positive for EGF receptor. This is based on the reliability of counting with the specific activity of EGF we use routinely.

Relationship of EGF receptor to Oestrogen Receptor

In our studies, we measured "nuclear" and "cytoplasmic" receptor in all primary tumours (Sainsbury et al., 1985). Although it is clear that oestrogen receptor (ER) is nuclear in location, there is a more easily extractable component, the "cytoplasmic receptor". In analyses we included tumours with either type of ER positivity as ER positive.

EGF receptor was detected in the range of 10–187 fmol/mg membrane protein. Two binding sites were identified by Scatchard analysis, the higher affinity having a kilodalton range of 0.17–2.9 nM. Steady-state binding was reached in 1 h at 26 °C and was similar to that observed at 37 °C.

In 228 primary tumours, there was a striking inverse correlation of EGF receptor with ER (Table 1) ($p < 0.0001$). For the purposes of statistical analysis, EGF binding < 10 fmol/mg membrane proteins was considered to be EGF receptor negative, and ER binding < 5 fmol/mg cytosol protein was ER negative. The ER-negative tumours can thus be split into two groups, those which are EGF receptor positive and those which are EGF receptor negative. The ligand binding results were compared with semiquantitative grading of EGF receptor by immunohistochemistry, and there was a significant correlation (Sainsbury et al., 1985). EGF receptor measured by ligand binding is more sensitive than immunochemistry, accounting for EGF receptor-positive tumours that are negative in histochemistry.

Table 1. EGF receptor in 228 primary breast carcinomas

		EGF receptor		
		Positive (n)	Negative (n)	Total (n)
ER	Positive	12	86	98
	Negative	68	62	130
		80	148	228

These results suggest that endogenous ligands are not interfering with the EGF receptor assay, since R_1 antibody reacts with a peptide-external domain of the EGF receptor and does not interfere with the binding site for EGF.

Failure to demonstrate EGF receptor on the majority of ER-positive tumours contrasts with in vitro work on the MCF-7 (ER-positive) human breast cancer cell line. They express a low level of EGF receptor, are stimulated to grow by EGF and produce transforming growth factor (TGF) alpha (Dickson et al., 1986). It is possible that low levels of EGF receptor in vivo in ER-positive tumours are further down-regulated by TGF-alpha and hence not detectable by ligand-binding studies. There is, however, a good correlation of immunohistochemical demonstration of EGF receptor with ligand binding, so high surface levels of EGF receptor occupied by locally secreted TGF-alpha would not account for the EGF receptor-negative tumours.

Correlation of EGF Receptor with Differentiation, Size of Tumour and Lymph Nodes

To correlate EGF receptor with other prognostic variables, Bloom and Richardson grading was carried out on 108 primary tumours (Table 2) (Sainsbury et al., 1985a). EGF receptors were correlated with poorly differentiated tumours. The inverse correlation of EGF receptor with ER also occurred in regional lymph node

Table 2. Correlation of Bloom and Richardson grading and EGF receptor

		I (n)	II (n)	III (n)	Total (n)
EGF receptor	Positive	2	11	32	45
	Negative	10	25	28	63
		12	36	60	108

$p < 0.002$.

Table 3. Relation between size of tumour and epidermal growth factor receptor state

	Size (cm)				
	<2 (n)	2.1–3.5 (n)	3.6–5 (n)	>5 (n)	Total (n)
Epidermal growth factor receptors:					
Positive	8	22	7	8	45
Negative	21	28	9	5	63
Total	29	50	16	13	108
Positive for epidermal growth factor receptors (%)	28	44	44	62	

λ^2 for logit-linear trend in proportions $= 3.97$ with 1 df; $p = 0.046$.

Table 4. Lymph node status and EGF receptor status

	EGF receptor positive (n)	EGF receptor negative (n)
Nodes clear	8	18
Nodes involved	25	20

metastases: Three ER-positive metastases were EGF receptor-negative and ten EGF receptor-negative metastases were ER-negative ($p < 0.02$). No EGF receptor-positive metastases arose from primary tumours that were EGF receptor-negative.

There was also a correlation of EGF receptor with increasing tumour size (Table 3). There were more EGF receptor-positive tumours in patients with involved regional lymph nodes (Table 4).

Are These Abnormal EGF Receptors?

None of the methods described above would detect EGF receptor analogous to erb-B, which lacks the external domain and shows much less autophosphorylation than EGF receptor. We therefore used a polyclonal antibody raised to a synthetic peptide homologous to a region of the internal EGF receptor domain (gift of W. Gullick). Forty-two primary tumours were studied. The particular immunochemical pattern that would show an erbB-type protein would be negative staining with R_1 antibody but positive staining with the internal antibody. The control for the internal antibody consisted of pre-incubation with the synthetic peptide to which it was raised. Only two tumours showed this pattern, and they were also EGF receptor negative by ligand binding. Unfortunately, there was insufficient material for molecular biological studies – so this remains to be confirmed. However, it is clear that this is not a common finding in breast cancer ($< 5\%$ of cases).

Cut-off Points for EGF Receptor-Positive Tumours

Three other groups have confirmed the reciprocal relationship of EGF receptors to ER, although in the case of Fitzpatrick et al. (1984) the results were not significant. Their EGF receptor values ranged from 1–121 fmol/ml membrane protein in 137 tumours. Perez *et al.* (1984) found a range of 1–64 fmol/mg membrane protein and a significant inverse relationship in 95 human breast cancers. The Kd mean was $3.7 \times 10^{-9} M$, and in pooled samples Fitzpatrick *et al.* (1984) found a value of 2 nM. Fabbro *et al.* (1986) found a range of 2–80 fmol/mg membrane protein and a significant inverse relationship with oestrogen receptor. Thus, a total of 500 breast tumours have been described with good agreement of Kd and binding capacity. However, the cut-off point for correlating EGF receptors with other variables is different in each series.

Since we have shown a highly significant association of EGF receptor status with ER-negative and poorly differentiated tumours, it would appear that our definition of EGF receptor positive can be justified on the grounds of both the usefulness of the clinical correlation and the analysis of counting reliability.

Prognostic Significance of EGF Receptor

The prognostic significance of EGF receptor status as defined above has now been analysed on the first 135 patients followed prospectively (Sainsbury et al., 1987). As expected, there is a slower relapse initially with ER-positive tumours but 3 years after initial diagnosis, the relapse-free survival (RFS) curves come together again. Nevertheless, the curves for RFS and overall survival (OS) are both significantly different for ER-positive and ER-negative tumours.

Of particular interest is the result for ER-negative tumours stratified by EGF receptor status. There is a highly significant difference in OS as well as RFS, with EGF receptor-positive patients having a much higher mortality. RFS is 76% versus 39% at 3 years, and OS is 82% versus 41%. The difference between ER-positive tumours and ER-negative EGF receptor-negative tumours is not significant. Thus, the early separation of survival curves for ER-negative and ER-positive tumours can be accounted for by the rapid demise of ER-negative EGF receptor-positive patients, and the coming together of the survival curves is related to the better prognosis of ER-negative EGF receptor-positive patients. These results provide an explanation for a major controversy in the literature on the effect of ER status on RFS. Studies following patients for over 5 years generally do not show a significant effect on RFS, but those analysing at 1–2 years do. An early relapsing, poor-prognosis subgroup would account for these results. We have defined such a subgroup by EGF receptor status.

There are other known prognostic factors such as tumour size and Bloom and Richardson grading, so we analysed these factors in our patients. There was no significant separation of survival (OS or RFS) using these criteria. Stratifying for these variables, EGF receptor-positive tumours always had the worst survival. Positive lymph node status and ER-negative tumours were associated with worse survival, but the patients with EGF receptor-positive tumours within a subgroup always had worse survival than those with EGF receptor-negative tumours.

The separation of a poor prognostic subgroup in a relatively low number of patients followed up for 3 years suggests that EGF receptor status is a powerful discriminator and could be used for prospective trials of adjuvant therapy.

The expression of EGF receptors and poor prognosis suggests that the initial hypothesis is correct that tumours expressing more EGF receptors could be more responsive to endogenous growth factors. This therefore provides new therapeutic options for this group of patients.

The Association of EGF Receptors and ER with Membrane-Bound Tissue Plasminogen Activator and Urokinase

To try and relate the expression of EGF receptors to other biological variables associated with aggressive tumour behaviour, we investigated plasminogen activators in the primary tumour membranes. Plasminogen activators (PA) are serine protease enzymes which initiate extracellular proteolysis by cleaving plasminogen to yield the active protease plasmin. The PA are involved in numerous physiological processes in which proteolysis is featured, such as tissue remodelling, regression of breast lobules. There is a large amount of evidence that the PA are also involved in tumour invasion and metastasis (reviewed in Dano et al., 1985).

Two types of PA are described, namely tissue plasminogen activator (tPA) and urokinase (uPA). They differ not only in molecular weight and immunologically but also in their function, and it is known that they are products of separate genes (Tripputi et al., 1986). tPA depends upon the presence of fibrin to achieve efficient activation of plasminogen, and so it is considered to be the main PA involved in fibrinolysis. Urokinase has no fibrin dependence and is associated with the regulation of extracellular proteolysis (Dano et al., 1985). Both types of PA have been identified in cancers.

The regulation of PA secretion is influenced by hormones in several cancer cell lines. Oestradiol stimulates PA secretion in MCF-7 (Butler et al., 1979), ZR75-1 (Huff and Lippmann, 1984) and UCT Br-1 (Wilson et al., 1982) breast cancer cell lines and EGF stimulates PA secretion in HeLa (Lee and Weinstein, 1978) and A431 (Gross et al., 1983) cells. An association between PA activity and ER concentration has been identified in human breast tumours (Duffy et al., 1986) but so far no work exists concerning the relationship between PA activity and EGF receptor in human tumours.

PA are strongly bound to cells, although they are also found in solution in many body fluids. The membrane-bound form may be of more significance than the soluble one, since it would block enzyme activity around the tumour. Inhibitors do not block bound urokinase. A membrane receptor for uPA has been described recently which binds uPA to the external surface of the cell in the active form (Vassalli et al., 1985). We have demonstrated that this receptor is present in breast cancers (Needham et al., 1987).

Because of in vitro evidence of hormonal regulation of different types of PA, and because membrane-bound PA may be of most biological relevance, we have investigated the occurrence of membrane-associated PA in 43 breast cancers and have studied its relationship to both ER and EGF receptor status.

The PA assay used fibrin as substrate to ensure that tPA activity was not underestimated, and antibodies to uPA and tPA were used to quench the activity of each PA type so that they could be measured separately.

Tumours were divided into ER-positive EGF receptor-negative ER-negative EGF receptor-negative and ER-negative EGF receptor-negative groups. While there was no significant difference in total PA and uPA between any group and another, tPA was significantly lower in ER-negative EGF receptor-positive tumours (Table 5). The ER-negative EGF receptor-negative tumours did not differ significantly from ER-positive EGF receptor-negative tumours. Therefore, ER status alone was not the major determinant of tPA, but a lack of ER but at the sometime the presence of EGF receptor was associated with low tPA levels.

Our present results are consistent with the findings of Duffy et al. (1986), who demonstrated a correlation between tPA and ER. ER-negative tumours possessed lower tPA activity than ER-positive tumours. Higher tPA levels in ER-positive tumours might also be expected, since oestrogens are known to stimulate tPA but

Table 5. Correlation of ER, EGF receptor, and PA

n	ER	EGF receptor	Total PA	tPA	uPA	%uPA
3	+	+	1948	777	255	7
12	+	−	2005	1132*	625	49**
10	−	+	1034	140*	826	87**
18	−	−	1030	384	475	55

+, positive; −, negative.
Log mean PA activity min uPA mg protein^{-1}.
$*p = 0.003$; $**p = 0.0004$.

not uPA secretion in the cell line MCF-7 (Ryan et al., 1984). The lack of tPA appears to be associated with an aggressive group of tumours, and it is possible that EGF receptors play a role in suppressing tPA secretion. Alternatively, they may be independent features in the phenotype of these tumours. Thorsen (1982) postulated that tumour cells arrested in circulation by microthrombi might free themselves if they were able to secrete PA. Since tPA is mostly concerned with fibrinolysis, this is one mechanism by which a lack of tPA may contribute to a more aggressive phenotype.

Conclusions

EGF receptors are of prognostic significance in breast cancer and help define a group of patients who will respond poorly to hormone therapy. They could be used for stratification for adjuvant trials and provide a target for new approaches to therapy.

References

Butler WB, Kirkland WL, Jorgensen TL (1979) Induction of plasminogen activator by estrogen in a human breast cancer cell line (MCF-7). Biochem Biophys Res Commun 90: 1328–1334

Carpenter G (1985) Binding assays for epidermal growth factor. Methods Enzymol 109: 101–110

Dano K, Andreasen PA, Grondahl-Hansen J, Kristensen P, Neilsen LS, Skriver L (1985) Plasminogen activators, tissue degradation and cancer. Adv Cancer Res 44: 139–226

Dickson RB, Bates SE, McManaway ME, Lippman ME (1986) Characterisation of estrogen responsive transforming activity in human breast cancer cell lines. Cancer Res 46: 1707–1713

Duffy MJ, O'Grady P, Simon J, Rose M, Lijnen HR (1986) Tissue type plasminogen activator in breast cancer: relationship with estradiol and progesterone receptors. J Natl Cancer Inst 77: 621–623

Fabbro D, Wyss R, Borner C, Regazzi R (1986) Epidermal growth factor receptor and calcium/phospholipid-dependent protein kinase activities in human mammary tumour cells. In: Eppenberger U, Fabbro D, Schäfer P (eds) Endocrine therapy of breast cancer, Karger, Basel, pp 33–44. Contribution to oncology, vol 23

Fitzpatrick SL, Brightwell J, Wittliff JL, Barrows GH, Schultz GS (1984) Epidermal growth factor binding by breast tumour biopsies and relationship to estrogen and progestin receptor levels. Cancer Res 44: 3448–3453

Gross JL, Krupp MN, Rifkin DB, Lane DM (1983) Down-regulation of epidermal growth factor receptor correlates with plasminogen activator activity in human A431 epidermoid carcinoma cells. Proc Natl Acad Sci USA 80: 2276–2280

Huff K, Lippmann ME (1984) Hormonal control of plasminogen activator secretion in ZR-75-1 human breast cancer cells in culture. Endocrinol 114: 1702–1710

Lee LS, Weinstein IB (1978) Epidermal growth factor-like phorbol esters induce plasminogen activator in HeLa cells. Nature 274: 696–697

Needham GK, Sherbet GV, Farndon JR, Harris AL (1987) Binding of urokinase to specific receptor sites on human breast cancer membranes. Br J Cancer 55: 13–16

Perez R, Pascual M, Macias A, Lage A (1984) Epidermal growth factor receptors in human breast cancer. Breast Cancer Res Treat 4: 189–193

Ryan TJ, Seeger JI, Kumar SA, Dickerman HW (1984) Estradiol preferentially enhances extracellular tissue plasminogen activators of MCF-7 breast cancer cells. J Biol Chem 259: 14324–14327

Sainsbury JRC, Malcolm AJ, Appleton DR, Farndon JR, Harris AL (1985a) Presence of epidermal growth factor receptor as an indicator of poor prognosis in patients with breast cancer. J Clin Pathol 38: 1225–1228

Sainsbury JRC, Farndon JR, Sherbet GV, Harris AL (1985b) Epidermal growth factor receptors and oestrogen receptors in human breast cancers. Lancet I: 364–366

Sainsbury JRC, Farndon JR, Needham GK, Malcolm AJ, Harris AL (1987) Epidermal growth factor receptor status as predictor of early recurrence of and death from breast cancer. Lancet I: 1398–1402

Thorsen T (1982) Association of plasminogen activator activity and steroid receptors in human breast cancers. Eur J Cancer Clin Oncol 18: 129–132

Tripputi P, Blasi F, Ny T, Emanuel BS, Lefofsky J, Croce CM (1986) Tissue type plasminogen activator gene is on chromosome 8. Cytogenet Cell Genet 42: 24–28

Vassalli JD, Baccino D, Belin D (1985) A cellular binding site for the Mr 55,000 form of the human plasminogen activator urokinase. J Cell Biol 100: 86–92

Wilson EL, Dutlow C, Dowdle EB (1982) Effect of hormones on the secretion of plasminogen activator by a new line of human breast carcinoma cells, UCT-Br1. In: Growth of Cells in Hormonally Defined Media. Cold Spring Harbor Laboratory, Cold Spring Harbor, New York, pp 849–854

The Transformation-Suppressive Function Is Lost in Tumorgenic Cells and Is Restored upon Transfer of a Suppressor Gene

E. Iten[1], A. Ziemiecki[2], and R. Schäfer[3]

Ludwig Institut für Krebsforschung, Inselspital, 3010 Bern, Switzerland
Present addresses:
[1] Zentrallaboratorium Blutspendedienst, SRK, Wankdorfstraße 10, 3022 Bern, Switzerland
[2] Institut für Klinische und Experimentelle Forschung, Tiefenauspital, 3004 Bern, Switzerland
[3] Abteilung für Krebsforschung, Institut für Pathologie, Universitätsspital Zürich, Schmelzbergstraße 12, 8091 Zürich, Switzerland

Introduction

Multiple genetic changes are involved in the conversion of a normal cell into a malignant cell. The nature of genetic alterations in tumor cells has been analyzed by DNA transfection experiments and dominantly acting cellular oncogenes have been identified. The introduction of single activated oncogenes into immortalized cell lines such as mouse NIH/3T3 cells is sufficient for tumorigenic transformation. The requirements for malignant transformation of nonimmortalized, diploid cells are more complex in as much as combinations of oncogenes (e.g. *ras* and *myc* genes) or overexpression of single oncogenes and additional genetic alterations are needed (for review see Bishop 1987). Cell-cell fusion experiments have shown that the normal phenotype is restored in somatic cell hybrids of tumorigenic cell lines and normal cells (suppression of malignancy, for review see Klein 1987; Sager 1986; Schäfer 1987). We have demonstrated that rat embryo fibroblasts which have often been used as recipient cells for the introduction of "dominant-acting" oncogenes are still capable of suppressing the neoplastic phenotype when fused with a H-*ras* transformed rat cell line. The neoplastic phenotype is re-expressed in hybrids which have lost chromosomes (Griegel et al. 1986). These results suggest that a tumor suppressor gene expressed in normal cells is able to counteract the neoplastic transformation induced by a *ras* gene and that the loss or inactivation of the suppressor gene is a prerequisite for the transforming activity of the oncogene.

To define the stage in the process of oncogene-induced tumorigenesis at which suppressor genes are inactivated, we assayed the transformation-suppressive function in nontumorigenic rat 208F cells, in H-*ras* transfected tumorigenic FE-8 cells, and in phenotypic revertants derived from the FE-8 cell line. Loss of anchorage requirement for growth was chosen as the parameter of neoplastic transformation. In the present study, we report that immortalized rat 208F cells are capable of suppressing neoplastic transformation upon fusion with cells transformed by retroviral oncogenes. The transformation-suppressive function of these cells can no longer be detected in FE-8 cells which are neoplastically transformed with an activated human H-*ras* gene. The introduction of a suppressor gene that we have recently isolated (Schäfer et al. 1988) resulted in the restoration of the transformation-suppressive function in *ras*-transformed cells. We conclude that suppressor gene activity is lost during neoplastic progression rather than upon immortalization.

Materials and Methods

Cell Culture and Isolation of Somatic Cell Hybrids

All cells were grown in Dulbecco's modified Eagle's medium containing 10% fetal calf serum, penicillin (100 units/ml), and streptomycin (100 μg/ml) (standard medium). To determine the ability of cell lines to proliferate without anchorage, 100–1000 cells were plated into semisolid agar medium (standard medium supplemented with 0.15% [wt/vol] Difco Noble agar (Schäfer et al. 1983). Colonies were scored 2–3 weeks later. For somatic cell hybridization, cells were cocultured in standard medium for 24 h. Cellular hybrids were isolated after polyethylene glycol fusion and selection in standard medium supplemented with HAT additives (100 μM hypoxanthine, 0.4 μM aminopterin, 16 μM thymidine; Littlefield 1964; Szybalska and Szybalski 1962) and hygromycin B (400 μg/ml) (selective medium) as described (Davis and Willecke 1977). Twenty-four hours after fusion, cells were trypsinized and plated into selective medium containing 0.15% (wt/vol) Difco Noble agar (selective semisolid agar medium). An aliquot of the cell suspension was maintained in monolayer cultures on plastic dishes without agar. Colonies of somatic cell hybrids in semisolid agar cultures and in monolayer cultures were counted after 2–3 weeks. Individual hybrid clones were isolated from monolayer cultures with the help of stainless steel cylinders and grown into mass cultures. The DNA content of parental cells and of somatic cell hybrids was determined by flow cytometric analysis as described (Griegel et al. 1986).

Plasmid Transfection

Cotransfection of plasmids pMV3/ASVsrc (DeLorbe et al. 1980) and pSV2gpt (Mulligan and Berg 1981) onto F9 cells was accomplished by calcium phosphate coprecipitation as described by Wigler et al. (1978). The plasmids pMV3/ASV src and pSV2gpt express the v-*src* oncogene and the bacterial gene coding for *Escherichia coli* xanthine-guanine phosphoribosyltransferase, respectively. A quantity of 10 μg pMV3/ASVsrc DNA was mixed with 1 μg of pSV2gpt DNA, coprecipitated and added to a 10-cm diameter Petri dish containing 5×10^5 F9 cells. Twenty-four hours after transfection, cells were trypsinized and replated onto five dishes. Selection in standard medium plus HAT additives was initiated 24 h later. Colonies of HAT-resistant transfectants were visible after 2 weeks.

Determination of pp60^{v-src} Kinase Activity

pp60^{v-src} kinase activity in somatic cell hybrids and transfectants was assayed by the procedure described by Collett and Erikson (1978) with modifications. pp60^{v-src} was immunoprecipitated from cell lysates using a tumor-bearing rabbit (TBR) serum. Cell extracts in phosphate-buffered saline containing 1% Triton X-100, 100 μM sodiumorthovanadate, and 2 mM EDTA, were incubated with an excess (typically 5 μl) of TBR serum for 1 h on ice. Immunocomplexes were isolated by incubation with protein A-containing *Staphylococcus aureus*. The suspension of bacteria-bound complexes was washed twice with lysis buffer and resuspended in the kinase reaction mixture containing 10 mM Tris-HCl, pH 7.3, 10 mM MnCl$_2$, 100 μM sodiumorthovanadate, and 5 μl γ-^{32}P ATP (specific activity > 5000 Ci/mmole). The reaction was incubated on ice for 15 min, the bacteria pelleted and resuspended in SDS-PAGE sample buffer, and boiled. Bacteria were removed by centrifugation and the supernatant loaded onto a 11% SDS/polyacrylamide gel. After electrophoresis, gels were dried and autoradiographed. The ^{32}P-labelled IgG heavy chains were excised and Cerenkov radiation counted to quantitate the incorporation of labelled ATP. Protein determinations in cell extracts were performed as described (Schaffner and Weissman 1973).

Results and Discussion

Loss of the Transformation-Suppressive Function in an Immortalized Rat Cell Line upon Introduction of an Activated Human H-ras Gene

All cell lines used in this study are described in Table 1. The established rat fibroblastoid cell line 208F-3 does not form tumors in newborn rats or nude mice and does not grow in semisolid agar medium. We isolated 208F-3 cells from the 208F cell line after transfection with the hygromycin B resistance gene *(hph)* (Blochlinger and Diggelmann 1984), and selection in a standard medium containing hygromycin B (HMB). The cell line is deficient in hypoxanthin phosphoribosyltransferase (EC 2.4.2.8). Therefore, HMB-resistant 208F-3 cells can be used as "universal hybridizers" in cell fusion experiments with any wild-type cell line. The selection of cells in HAT medium (Littlefield 1964; Szybalska and Szybalski 1962) containing HMB allows the survival of somatic cell hybrids only.

We fused 208F-3 cells with tumorigenic NIH/3T3 cells transformed by the v-H-*ras* (NIHpZSR-11), the v-*src* (NIH 90 src), and the v-*fgr* oncogene (NIH GR-3) and with NIH/3T3 cells transformed by Polyoma virus (NIH Po-8a). After fusion, the cells were plated into selective medium containing 0.15% (wt/vol) agar, thus allowing the growth of transformed, anchorage-independent hybrid colonies only. To assay the efficiency of cell fusion, an aliquot of the cells was plated on plastic culture dishes in selective medium without agar. The results of the cell fusion experiments are summarized in Table 2. Hybrid populations of 208F-3 cells and NIH/3T3 cells transformed by v-Ha-*ras*, v-*src*, and v-*fgr* oncogenes were unable to proliferate in selective semisolid agar medium. We conclude from these results that immortalized 208F-3 cells have retained the ability to suppress the an-

Table 1. Cell lines used in this study

Designation	Origin	Efficiency of cloning (%)	
		In semisolid agar culture	In monolayer culture
208F-3	HMB-resistant clone derived from rat 208F cells (Quade 1979), HPRT$^-$	<0.01	not determined
FE-8Y	HMB-resistant clone derived from rat FE-8 cells. Tumorigenic FE-8 cells were isolated from 208F cells after cotransfection of the activated human H-*ras* gene (Tabin et al. 1982) and pSV2neo (Southern and Berg 1982), HPRT$^-$	49	44
NIHpZSR-11	Tumorigenic clone of NIH/3T3 cells infected with a recombinant retrovirus harboring the v-H-*ras* and neo genes (Redmond et al. 1988), HPRT$^+$	26	80
NIH 90 src	NIH/3T3 cells infected with the temperature-sensitive avian sarcoma virus (ASV) mutant LA 90 (Hunter et al. 1979), HPRT$^+$	71	62
NIH GR-3	A clone of NIH/3T3 cells grown in agar medium derived from a cell population transfected with pGR (Naharro et al. 1983), a plasmid containing feline sarcoma virus (Gardner Rasheed strain), HPRT$^+$	24	not determined
NIH Po-8a	NIH/3T3 cells infected with Polyoma virus, HPRT$^+$	0.5	34
FSC-2	A clone of 208F cells grown in agar medium derived from cells cotransfected with plasmids pMV3/ASVsrc (DeLorbe et al. 1980) and pSV2gpt (Mulligan and Berg 1981), resistant to HAT medium	79	63
FSC-3	Morphologically transformed cell clone derived from 208F cells as FSC-2, resistant to HAT medium	21	51
F9	HMB-resistant phenotypic revertant derived from tumorigenic FE-8 cells (Schäfer et al. 1988), HPRT$^-$	<0.1	60
NIH/3T3	Nontumorigenic mouse cell line, HPRT$^+$	<0.1	not determined

HAT medium, standard medium supplemented with hypoxanthine, aminopterin and thymidine, as described in "Materials and Methods"; *HMB*, hygromycin B; *HPRT$^-$*, cells deficient in hypoxanthin phosphoribosyltransferase, sensitive to HAT medium; *HPRT$^+$*, wild type cells, resistant to HAT medium.

Table 2. Suppression of anchorage-independent proliferation in cellular hybrid populations

Hybrid cells	Hybrid frequency $\times 10^{-3}$	Agar$^+$ hybrid frequency $\times 10^{-3}$	Ratio of agar$^+$ hybrids to total hybrid frequency
Fusions involving immortalized nontumorigenic 208F-3 cells			
208F-3 × NIH/3T3	3	<0.01	<0.003
208F-3 × NIHpZSR-11	2.3	<0.01	<0.004
208F-3 × NIH 90 src	0.8	<0.01	<0.01
208F-3 × NIH GR-3	2.1	<0.01	<0.004
208F-3 × NIH Po-8a	8.7	0.23	0.03
Fusions involving H-*ras* transformed 208F cells			
FE-8Y × NIH/3T3	2.1	0.43	0.2
FE-8Y × NIHpZSR-11	1.5	0.44	0.3
FE-8Y × NIH 90 src	1.7	1.2	0.7
FE-8Y × NIH GR-3	2.0	1.7	0.85
FE-8Y × NIH Po-8a	3.9	0.9	0.23
Fusions involving F9 revertants			
F9 × NIH/3T3	2.0	<0.01	<0.005
F9 × NIHpZSR-11	1.2	0.1	0.08
F9 × NIH 90 src	1.0	0.01	0.01
F9 × FSC-3	1.8	<0.01	<0.006
F9 × FSC-2	2.4	<0.01	<0.004
F9 × NIH GR-3	2.0	0.13	0.065
F9 × NIH Po-8a	4.3	0.12	0.03

chorage-independent proliferation of transformed cells. A significant proportion of cell hybrids between Polyoma-virus–transformed NIH/3T3 cells and 208F-3 cells were anchorage-independent. Since the cloning efficiency in semisolid agar medium of transformed parental cells was relatively low (0.5%, cf. Table 1), we conclude that anchorage-independent proliferation is not significantly reduced in 208F-3 × NIH Po-8a hybrids (Relative cloning efficiency of hybrid population: 2.8%). Somatic cell hybrids between nontumorigenic NIH/3T3 cells and *ras*-transformed 208F cells (FE-8Y, cf. Table 1) were anchorage-independent. Thus, in contrast to rat 208F-3 cells, mouse NIH/3T3 cells have lost the transformation-suppressive function.

Next we analyzed the expression of the neoplastic phenotype in somatic cell hybrids between H-*ras*-transformed 208F cells and the transformed NIH/3T3 cell lines. Tumorigenic FE-8Y cells were obtained after transfection of an activated human H-*ras* gene into 208F cells (Griegel et al. 1986) and subsequent introduction of the *hph* gene. Somatic cell hybrids of FE-8Y cells and NIH/3T3 cell lines transformed by the v-H-*ras* (NIHp25R-11), the v-*src* (NIH 90 src), or the v-*fgr* oncogene (NIH GR-3) and by Polyoma virus (NIH Po-8a) exhibited unrestricted growth in selective semisolid agar medium. We assume that the transformation-suppressive function has been lost during transfection of 208F cells by an activated human H-*ras* gene and selection of a clonal population of malignant cells. However, if the suppressor gene activity is sufficient to inhibit neoplastic transfor-

mation induced by one oncogene, the unrestricted function of the second oncogene present in the somatic cell hybrids will suffice for anchorage-independent
proliferation. Therefore, expression of the neoplastic phenotype in somatic cell
hybrids of *ras*-transformed FE-8Y cells and transformed NIH/3T3 cells does not
directly prove that a suppressor gene has been lost or inactivated following incorporation of an activated H-*ras* gene.

Restoration of the Transformation-Suppressive Function in a Phenotypic Revertant Derived from ras-Transformed Cells

The transformation-suppressive function was re-established in clone F9, a phenotypic revertant derived from FE-8 cells. This clone expresses a high amount of the
H-*ras*-encoded oncoprotein as determined by Western blot analysis of crude
membrane extracts with a *ras*-specific antibody. DNA prepared from F9 cells ex-
hibits transforming activity in an NIH/3T3 transfection assay. In spite of the continuous expression and biological activity of the H-*ras* oncogene, F9 cells have a
normal fibroblast-like morphology, require anchorage for growth and show a low
tumorigenicity in nude mice (Schäfer et al. 1988). Phenotypic reversion of F9 cells
is due to the incorporation of a human suppressor gene. Very recently, we have described the partial reversion of the transformed phenotype in FE-8 cells by gene
transfer (Schäfer et al. 1988). H-*ras*-transformed FE-8 cells were transfected with
human placenta DNA. All transfectants expressing the transformed phenotype
were selectively killed by treatment with the cardiac glycoside ouabain. *Ras*-trans-
formed cells are sensitive toward treatment with this drug, whereas normal cells
exhibit a relative resistance (Noda et al. 1983). Ouabain selection of the transfected FE-8 cell population resulted in the isolation of rare transfectants, including
F9, with a more normal phenotype. The normal phenotype was transferred onto
FE-8 cells in a second transfection cycle using F9 DNA as the donor. The human
DNA sequence that confers suppression of the neoplastic phenotype on FE-8 cells
has been molecularly cloned and the suppressor gene activity localized to an 18 kb
BamHI fragment (Schäfer et al. 1988).

Somatic cell fusion of F9 cells with three different cell lines transformed by the
v-*src* oncogene (NIH 90 src, FSC-2, FSC-3) resulted in hybrids that had lost the
ability to proliferate in semisolid agar medium (Table 2). The majority of the hybrids between F9 cells and NIHpZSR-11 cells (v-H-*ras* transformed NIH/3T3
cells) and of the hybrids between F9 and NIH GR-3 cells (v-*fgr* transformed
NIH/3T3 cells) were anchorage-dependent (Table 2). The relative cloning efficien-
cies of hybrid populations in agar medium were significantly reduced, when compared with transformed parental cells (cf. Table 1, hybrids of F9 and NIHpZSR-11
lines: 8%; hybrids of F9 and NIH GR-3 lines: 6.5%).

The relative cloning efficiency of a hybrid population isolated after fusion of F9
cells and NIH Po-8a cells was increased (2.8%) when compared with the parental
Polyoma virus-transformed cells (0.5%). We conclude from these results that F9
cells, similar to 208F-3 cells, were unable to suppress neoplastic transformation induced by Polyoma virus.

Genome Instability in Hybrids of ras-Resistant Revertants and src-Transformed Cells

The suppression of the neoplastic phenotype was analyzed not only in mass populations of somatic cell hybrids, but also in individual hybrid clones obtained from
an independent cell fusion experiment. Twenty-seven hybrid clones were isolated
after fusion of suppression-competent F9 cells with v-*src*-transformed FSC-2 and
FSC-3 cells (cf. Table 1 for a description of these cells). In a parallel experiment,

Table 3. Anchorage requirement in individual somatic cell hybrid clones and transfectants

Cells	Cloning efficiency in semisolid agar medium (%)	Cloning efficiency in standard medium in surfaces (%)
Somatic cell hybrids F9 × FSC-3		
FC3-1	0.1	54
FC3-2	0.8	30
FC3-3	<0.1	46
FC3-4	0.6	39
FC3-6	8.7	30
FC3-7	<0.1	54
FC3-8	<0.1	28
FC3-9	<0.1	68
FC3-10	27	58
FC3-11	0.5	53
FC3-12	0.2	33
FC3-13	<0.1	24
FC3-14	0.3	63
FC3-15	0.2	55
FC3-16	<0.1	68
FC3-17	0.2	56
FC3-18	0.4	36
FC3-19	2.7	45
FC3-20	<0.1	25
FC3-21	0.5	45
FC3-22	2.6	28
FC3-23	9.4	48
FC3-24	7.2	54
Somatic cell hybrids F9 × FSC-2		
FC2-1	2.7	58
FC2-2	0.9	46
FC2-3	4.4	35
FC2-4	1.0	38
F9 transfectants		
F9 src A2	4	6
F9 src A4	3	9
F9 src B1	1.5	8
F9 src B2	<0.1	not determined
F9 src B4	2	10
F0 src C1	3.5	12
F9 src C5	2.5	6

Table 4. pp60^{v-src} Kinase activity in somatic cell hybrids and transfectants

	Incorporation of γ-^{32}P-labeled ATP (fmol/mg protein)
Parental cells	
FSC-3	1.0
Somatic cell hybrids F9 × FSC-3	
FC3-3	0.04
FC3-4	0.05
FC3-8	0.03
FC3-10	0.4
FC3-12	0.14
FC3-14	0.07
FC3-16	0.11
FC3-17	0.23
F9 transfectants	
F9 src A2	2.6
F9 src A4	2.2
F9 src B1	2.2
F9 src C5	3.1

the v-*src* oncogene was introduced into F9 cells by transfection. Seven F9 subclones were isolated after cotransfection of the plasmids pMV3/ASVsrc (DeLorbe et al. 1980) and pSV2gpt (Mulligan and Berg 1981). Of the 27 hybrid clones, 19 exhibited poor or no growth in semisolid agar medium (Table 3). The activity of the v-*src* oncogene was analyzed in cellular hybrids and neoplastically transformed transfectants by determining pp60^{v-src} kinase activity in crude cell extracts. The anchorage-independent phenotype was expressed in one hybrid clone with the highest kinase activity (corresponding to 25% of the activity found in v-*src*-transformed parental FSC-3 cells: see Table 4). Seven hybrid clones exhibited low kinase activity (less than 12.5% of the level found in parental cells) and showed only poor growth in agar medium (cloning efficiency less than 0.6%).

The down-regulation of v-*src* expression in hybrids exhibiting anchorage requirement for growth is probably not due to suppressor gene activity. To analyze the persistence of integrated v-*src* copies in somatic cell hybrids, DNA was prepared from hybrid clones, digested with different restriction enzymes, and subjected to Southern blot analysis using a v-*src*-specific DNA probe. In all somatic cell hybrids that exhibited the normal phenotype, DNA fragments detected by this probe were different from those identified in the parental v-*src*-transformed cells (data not shown) indicating structural DNA rearrangements in the hybrids of F9 and FSC-2 or FSC-3 cells. Thus, further analysis of the mechanisms of suppression of anchorage-independent proliferation in individual hybrid clones is hampered by the inherent instability of hybrid genomes.

F9 cells transfected with pMV3/ASV src formed colonies in semisolid agar medium (Table 3) and exhibited a more than twofold kinase activity when compared with v-*src*-transformed parental cells FSC-3 (Table 4). This suggests to us that the transfected tyrosine kinase oncogene is overexpressed in F9 transfectants and can probably overrule the effect of the suppressor gene.

The Transformation-Suppressive Function is Lost During Neoplastic Progression

Our results suggest that the transformation-suppressive function is retained in immortalized rat fibroblasts. Somatic cell hybrids between immortalized nontumorigenic 208F-3 cells and anchorage-independent NIH/3T3 cells transformed by v-*src*, v-*fgr*, or v-H-*ras* oncogenes required anchorage for growth (suppression of anchorage-independence). On introduction of an activated H-*ras* gene into 208F cells, the transformation-suppressive function can no longer be observed. On reversion of H-*ras*-transformed FE-8 cells due to the incorporation of a suppressor gene, the transformation-suppressive function is re-established in spite of the continuous expression of the oncogene (revertant clone F9). We propose that the suppressor gene introduced into clone F9 (Schäfer et al. 1988) replaces an endogenous suppressor gene that was still functionally active in 208F cells but was inactivated or lost in FE-8 cells. The ability of F9 revertants to suppress v-*src*-induced transformation is the same as that of nontumorigenic 208F cells. Suppression of soft agar growth was further demonstrated in most somatic cell hybrids of F9 cells and NIH/3T3 cells transformed by the v-H-*ras* and the v-*fgr* oncogene. The expression of the neoplastic phenotype in some of the hybrids is probably due to a gene dosage effect. Somatic cell hybrids of F9 cells and NIHpZSR-11 cells initially contain at least five copies of the activated *ras* genes, as inferred from the copy number in parental cells (Griegel et al. 1986; Schäfer et al. 1988; Redmond et al. 1988). Transfection of F9 cells with a v-*src* plasmid resulted in colonies of transformed cells exhibiting a high $pp60^{v-src}$ kinase activity. It is likely that the neoplastic phenotype can no longer be suppressed in these transfectants.

The transformation-suppressive function is a constant characteristic of normal diploid rodent fibroblasts with a finite life span (Griegel et al. 1986; Schäfer et al. 1983; other references reviewed by Sager 1986; Schäfer 1987). Immortalized, nontumorigenic cell lines have been shown to be heterogeneous with regard to this property. Suppressor activity has been demonstrated in a Chinese hamster cell line, CHEF/18, (Craig and Sager 1985), Swiss 3T3 cells (Marshall 1980), and Syrian hamster cell lines (Koi and Barrett 1986). Dyson et al. (1982) have reported that the rat cell line, Rat-1, from which 208F cells have been derived, lacks the suppressive function when fused with ASV-transformed cells. In contrast to this, the same authors found that B2E2 Rat-1 cells, another derivative of Rat-1, were able to suppress morphological transformation in somatic hybrids with v-*src*-transformed cells. The difference between Rat-1 cells and 208F or B2E2 cells may reflect the variability within a heterogeneous cell population. Of particular interest is the question as to whether NIH/3T3 cells have suppressing activity. Preneoplastic mouse NIH/3T3 cells have often been used as "normal" recipient cells in DNA transfection experiments using DNA from tumor cells as the donor. Cellular transforming genes of the *ras* family and oncogenes not related to *ras* have been identified and functionally characterized by this method (see Bishop 1987 for a review). Our results suggest that, unlike 208F cells, aneuploid NIH/3T3 fibroblasts have lost the suppressive function probably during establishment from primary cells or during maintenance in culture. Immortalized REF52 cells are refractory to neoplastic transformation by *ras* oncogenes (Franza et al. 1986). Koi and Barrett (1986) have shown that the tumor-suppressive function of established cell lines of Syrian hamster origin is gradually lost during neoplastic progression. However, the loss of suppressor gene activity can be analyzed by somatic cell hybridization experiments only in an indirect way. Further characterization of the molecularly ,cloned human suppressor gene (Schäfer et al. 1988) and its rat homologue will allow the direct assay of the structure and expression of transformation-suppressing genes in normal human cells, tumor x normal hybrids and in primary, established nontumorigenic and tumorigenic rat cells.

Suppression of the neoplastic phenotype with the continuous expression of an activated H-*ras* gene has been demonstrated in somatic cell hybrids between transformed Chinese hamster cells and a normal Chinese hamster cell line (Craig and Sager 1985), in rat FE-8 cells fused with normal rat embryo fibroblasts (Griegel et al. 1986), and in hybrids of EJ bladder carcinoma and normal human fibroblasts (Geiser et al. 1986). *Ras* expression in these suppressed hybrids was not or only slightly reduced when compared with tumorigenic parental cells. Incorporation of the molecularly cloned suppressor gene into FE-8 cells does not result in a down-regulation of oncogene expression (Schäfer et al. 1988). The suppressor gene appears to act either at a distant step in the *ras*-signalling pathway or in a *ras*-independent cellular pathway. In contrast to the suppressed derivatives of *ras*-transformed cells, oncogene activity was diminished in the suppressed somatic cell hybrids between ASV-transformed rat cells and uninfected Swiss/3T3 mouse cells (Marshall 1980; Dyson et al. 1982). Untransformed hybrids showed a decrease in viral RNA and pp60^{v-src} kinase activity. Smith et al. (1986) have shown that microinjection of an anti-*ras* monoclonal antibody into NIH/3T3 cells transformed by v-*src*, v-*fes*, and v-*fms* oncogene cells resulted in morphological reversion and reduction in ^{3}H-labelled thymidine incorporation, suggesting that c-*ras* proteins are essential for the maintenance of the transformed phenotype induced by these oncogenes. The suppression of neoplastic transformation in somatic cell hybrids of F9 cells and three different v-*src*-transformed cell lines suggests that the suppressor gene active in these revertants functions in a pathway that is common for the *ras* and *src* oncogenes. Further evidence for the existence of common biochemical pathways for transformation induced by *ras* and *src* oncogenes comes from the study of revertants obtained after mutagenesis of transformed cells. These cells have acquired mutations in cellular effector genes causing a block in the expression of the neoplastic phenotype in the presence of a functional oncogene. Flat revertants isolated from Kirsten murine sarcoma virus-transformed NIH/3T3 cells were resistant to retransformation by tyrosine kinase oncogenes v-*fes* and v-*src* (Noda et al. 1983). An anchorage-dependent revertant clone derived from mink cells transformed by the Gardner-Arnstein strain of Feline Sarcoma Virus was refractory to retransformation by retroviruses harboring the v-*fes*, v-*fms*, or v-*ras* oncogenes (Haynes and Downing 1988). The pattern of resistance was not always identical in these revertants, suggesting the existence of different biochemical pathways of transformation: Revertants that were resistent toward v-*fos*, v-*abl*, v-*mos*, and v-H-*ras* transformation could be retransformed by Polyoma middle T antigen and the *trk* oncogene coding for a tyrosine kinase (Zarbl et al. 1988).

Acknowledgements. We gratefully acknowledge the help of our colleagues who provided us with cell lines. NIH GR-3 cells were obtained from S. Kozma, Basel; NIH Po-8a cells from R. Müller, Marburg; NIHpZSR-11 cells from S. M. S. Redmond, Bern; and NIH 90 src cells from R. R. Friis, Bern. We are indebted to B. Groner for generously supporting our work.

References

Bishop JM (1987) The molecular genetics of cancer. Science 237: 305-311

Blochlinger K, Diggelmann H (1984) Hygromycin B phosphotransferase as a selectable marker for DNA transfer experiments with higher eucaryotic cells. Mol Cell Biol 4: 2929-2931

Collett MS, Erikson RL (1978) Protein kinase activity associated with the avian sarcoma virus src gene product. Proc Natl Acad Sci USA 75: 2012-2024

Craig R, Sager R (1985) Suppression of tumorigenicity in hybrids of normal and oncogene-transformed CHEF cells. Proc Natl Acad Sci USA 82: 2062-2066

Davies PJ, Willecke K (1977) Segregation of human hypoxanthine phosphoribosyltransferase activity from somatic cell hybrids isolated after fusion of mouse gene transfer cells with Chinese hamster cells. MGG 154: 191-197

DeLorbe WJ, Luciw PA, Goodman HM, Varmus HE, Bishop JM (1980) Molecular cloning and characterization of avian sarcoma virus circular DNA molecules. J Virol 36: 50-61

Dyson PJ, Quade K, Wyke JA (1982) Expression of the ASV src gene in hybrids between normal and virally transformed cells: Specific suppression occurs in some hybrids but not others. Cell 30: 491-498

Franza BR jr, Maruyama K, Garrels JI, Ruley HE (1986) In vitro establishment is not a sufficient prerequisite for transformation by activated ras oncogenes. Cell 44: 409-418

Geiser AG, Der CH, Marshall CJ, Stanbridge EJ (1986) Suppression of tumorigenicity with continuous expression of the c-Ha-ras oncogene in EJ bladder carcinoma-human fibroblast hybrids. Proc Natl Acad Sci USA 83: 5209-5213

Griegel D, Traub O, Willecke K, Schäfer R (1986) Suppression and reexpression of transformed phenotype in hybrids of Ha-ras 1 transformed Rat-1 cells and early passage rat embryo fibroblasts. Int J Cancer 38: 697-705

Haynes JR, Downing JR (1988) A recessive cellular mutation in v-fes-transformed mink cells restores contact inhibition and anchorage-dependent growth. Mol Cell Biol 8: 2419-2427

Hunter T, Sefton BM, Beemon K (1979) Studies on the structure and function of the avian sarcoma virus transforming-gene product. Symposia on Quantitative Biology, vol 44. Cold Spring Harbor Laboratories, Cold Spring Harbor, New York, pp 931-941

Klein G (1987) The approaching era of the tumor suppressor genes. Science 238: 1539-1545

Koi M, Barrett JC (1986) Loss of tumor-suppressive function during chemically induced neoplastic progression of Syrian hamster embryo cells. Proc Natl Acad Sci USA 83: 5992-5996

Littlefield JW (1964) Selection of hybrids from matings of fibroblasts in vitro and their presumed recombinants. Science 145: 709-710

Marshall CJ (1980) Suppression of the transformed phenotype with retention of the viral "src" gene in cell hybrids between Rous sarcoma virus-transformed rat cells and untransformed mouse cells. Exp Cell Res 127: 373-384

Mulligan RC, Berg P (1981) Selection for animal cells that express the *Escherichia coli* gene coding for xanthine-guanine phosphoribosyltransferase. Proc Natl Acad Sci 78: 2072–2076

Naharro G, Tronick SR, Rasheed S, Gardner MB, Aaronson SA, Robbins KC (1983) Molecular cloning of integrated Gardner-Rasheed feline sarcoma virus: Genetic structure of its cell-derived sequence differs from that of other tyrosine kinase-coding onc genes. J Virol 47: 611–619

Noda M, Selinger Z, Scolnick EM, Bassin RH (1983) Flat revertants isolated from Kisten sarcoma virus-transformed cells are resistant to the action of specific oncogenes. Proc Natl Acad Sci USA 80: 5602–5606

Quade K (1979) Transformation of mammalian cells by avian myelocytomatosis virus and avian erythroblastosis virus. Virology 98: 461–465

Redmond SMS, Friis RR, Reichmann E, Müller RG, Groner B, Hynes NE (1988) The transformation of primary and established mouse mammary epithelial cells by p21-*ras* is concentration-dependent. Oncogene 2: 259–265

Sager R (1986) Genetic suppression of tumor formation: A new frontier in cancer research. Cancer Res 46: 1573–1580

Schäfer R (1987) Suppression of the neoplastic phenotype and "anti-oncogenes". Blut 54: 257–265

Schäfer R, Hoffmann H, Willecke K (1983) Suppression of tumorigenicity in somatic cell hybrids of tumorigenic Chinese hamster cells and diploid mouse fibroblasts: Dependence on the presence of at least three different mouse chromosomes and independence of hamster genome dosage. Cancer Res 43: 2240–2246

Schäfer R, Iyer J, Iten E, Nirkko AC (1988) Partial reversion of the transformed phenotype in HRAS-transfected tumorigenic cells by transfer of a human gene. Proc Natl Acad Sci USA 85: 1590–1594

Schaffner W, Weissmann C (1973) A rapid, sensitive, and specific method for the determination of protein in dilute solution. Anal Biochem 56: 502–514

Smith MR, DeGudicibus, Stacey DW (1986) Requirement for c-*ras* proteins during viral oncogene transformation. Nature 320: 540–543

Southern PJ, Berg P (1982) Transformation of mammalian cells to antibiotic resistance with a bacterial gene under control of the SV40 early region promoter. J Mol Appl Genet 1: 327–341

Szybalska EH, Szybalski W (1962) Genetics of human cell lines: IV. DNA-mediated heritable transformation of a biochemical trait. Proc Natl Acad Sci USA 48: 2026–2034

Tabin CJ, Bradley SM, Bargmann CI, Weinberg RA, Papageorge AG, Scolnick EM, Dhar R, Lowy DR, Chang EH (1982) Mechanism of activation of a human oncogene. Nature 300: 143–149

Wigler M, Pellicer A, Silverstein S, Axel R (1978) Biochemical transfer of single-copy eukaryotic genes using total cellular DNA as donor. Cell 14: 725–731

Zarbl H, Latreille J, Jolicoeur P (1988) Revertants of v-*fos*-transformed fibroblasts have mutations in cellular genes essential for transformation by other oncogenes. Cell 51: 357–369

Subject Index